Getting Preg
A Guide for the Infer

Comments from the Press

Simply worded, easy to read and understand.... If fate has put infertility in your lot, do not feel helpless, just sit down, hold your partner's hand and together go through this book.... This book can also help general practitioners plan a more systematic approach towards infertility.

The Hindustan Times

A commendable work, this book is written lucidly and produced attractively.... Recommended for all infertile couples.

Indian Express

One of the most scientifically explained and comprehensively written books to instil hope among infertile couples who have lost all hope of having a baby.... A bible for infertile couples.

The Tribune

Offers information in a simple, straightforward fashion that is easy to understand. A must not only for all newly married couples but for their parents also.

Indian Review of Books

Getting Pregnant
A Guide for the Infertile Couple

Dr Aniruddha Malpani
Dr Anjali Malpani
Mrs Anne de Braganca Cunha

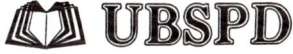

UBS Publishers' Distributors Ltd.
New Delhi ● Bombay ● Bangalore ● Madras ●
Calcutta ● Patna ● Kanpur ● London

UBS Publishers' Distributors Ltd.
5 Ansari Road, New Delhi-110 002
Mumbai Bangalore Madras Calcutta Patna Kanpur London

© Dr Aniruddha Malpani, Dr Anjali Malpani and
Anne de Braganca Cunha

First Published	1994
First Reprint	1994
Second Reprint	1995
Third Reprint	1996

All rights reserved. No part of this publication may be reproduced or transmitted in any form or by any means, electronic or mechanical including photocopying, recording, or any information storage and retrieval system, without permission in writing from the publisher.

Cover Design : UBS Art Studio
Cover Photograph : Fawzan Husain
Cartoons : Dr Hemant Morparia

Typeset at UBSPD in 11 pt. New Century Schoolbook
Printed at Rajkamal Electric Press, Delhi

To our parents, who made it all possible
To our patients, who are our inspiration
To our children, who make it all worthwhile

Preface

Grappling with infertility is very similar to finding yourself trapped in a complex maze. You can't see clearly what's ahead of you so you have no way of keeping your perspective. You wander the same path over and over again – totally lost and bewildered. You feel that you are all alone with no one to show you the way out.

There are many questions pertaining to infertility, but few answers. Who are the best doctors? Which is the most effective treatment? What options can be utilized so that the way out can be found?

The contents of this book are designed to provide infertile couples with a comprehensive picture of the infertility experience, in order to help them to negotiate their way through the maze as efficiently as possible. You need to find your own path – and this book will serve as a guide.

Infertility is a problem that affects both the man and the woman. It engenders feelings of fear, anxiety, anger, guilt, grief and, in the end, hope. It's a problem that reaches deep into your emotional life and invades your intimate relationships. Infertility can snatch away all your energy and concentration. This disorder can also demand a great deal of time and money and total commitment. It may become your life's obsession!

Confronting your infertility problem is a process that must be worked through carefully – it takes a good deal of both time and effort. This book will show you that infertility can be a difficult condition, but it will also provide you with ways and means of coping with and resolving this problem effectively.

The most important message that this book seeks to convey is that you *must* be an active participant in your medical treatment. You are a vital member of your medical team – the more you understand, the better you can participate in the decisions that directly affect your life. Infertility can bring about a feeling of helplessness because you cannot have a baby when you want to. An important way of regaining control of the situation is by taking an active part in resolving your infertility problem by being well informed.

Why is it so important that you be well informed? Unfortunately, many infertile couples have had unhappy experiences, due to lack of information. For instance:

1. They may have a problem for which there may be an effective treatment, but they may not be receiving this treatment. The kind of infertility for which there is no effective treatment is devastating, but infertility which can be and is not correctly treated is the real tragedy !
2. They may not have had the correct diagnosis made.
3. Their doctor – no matter how knowledgeable – may not be putting all the pieces together correctly for them.
4. They may be receiving treatment that is actually decreasing their chances of conceiving.
5. There is a certain tolerance limit which everyone has – and this limit may be financial, physical or emotional. Sometimes their tolerance limit may be exceeded before they receive appropriate treatment.

Most importantly, having the relevant information may make a difference in your getting pregnant. Such information can help you determine if your time, effort and money are being well spent. It can also help you to know when to quit trying. An informed approach will allow you to maintain control of your life, and will also help you realize that everything within your control has been done. And even if you don't get pregnant, you will at least feel satisfied that you fully understand your condition, and that you did your best to achieve your goal. That knowledge will be your strength.

This book can be read through from cover to cover – or you may choose to refer to just a particular chapter, pertaining to your specific problem. We have deliberately allowed some repetition, so that each chapter can stand on its own.

It is definitely not the purpose of this book to teach couples to bypass the medical care that they may need. On the contrary, the goal is to educate couples sufficiently so that they can find the right doctor and, as informed patients, participate effectively in their own care.

Our experience has been that the best patients are the well-informed ones – patients who take an active part in their own treatment, so that they can work with their doctor to develop an effective treatment plan. We hope this book helps in empowering infertile patients with the right information and knowledge so that they can make the right decisions for themselves! Finally, all the best to you in your quest for a baby!

Dr Aniruddha Malpani
Dr Anjali Malpani
Anne de Braganca Cunha

Contents

	Preface	vii
1.	How Babies are Made – The Basics	1
2.	Do You Have an Infertility Problem? When to Start Worrying	17
3.	Finding Out What's Wrong – The Basic Medical Tests	24
4.	Testing the Man: Semen Analysis	28
5.	Beyond the Semen Analysis	34
6.	Diagnosis and Treatment of Male Infertility – More Confusion!	42
7.	The Case of the Man with a Low Sperm Count	57
8.	Ultrasound – Seeing with Sound	61
9.	Laparoscopy – The Kinder Cut	67
10.	Hysteroscopy	76
11.	The Tubal Connection	80
12.	Ovulation – Normal and Abnormal	91
13.	Polycystic Ovarian Disease (PCOD)	103
14.	The Cervical Factor	106
15.	Hirsutism – Excess Facial and Body Hair	113
16.	Endometriosis – The Silent Invader	118
17.	Ectopic Pregnancy	124
18.	Unexplained Infertility	129
19.	Secondary Infertility – Caught between Fertile and Infertile Worlds	133

20.	Empty Arms – The Lonely Trauma of Miscarriage	**136**
21.	Understanding Your Medicines	**148**
22.	Artificial Insemination by the Husband's Sperm	**162**
23.	Test Tube Babies – IVF and GIFT	**169**
24.	Using Donor Sperm	**193**
25.	Surrogate Mothering	**201**
26.	When Enough Is Enough – The Decision to End Treatment	**205**
27.	Adoption – Yours by Choice	**210**
28.	Child-free Living – Life without Children	**217**
29.	The Emotional Crisis of Infertility	**223**
30.	How to Cope with Infertility	**230**
31.	Infertility and Sexuality	**241**
32.	Support Groups – Self-Help Is the Best Help	**248**
33.	Myths and Misconceptions about Infertility	**252**
34.	Helping Hands – How Friends and Relatives Can Help	**257**
35.	Making Decisions about Treatment	**260**
36.	Your Role on the Medical Team	**267**
37.	The Ethical Issues – Right or Wrong?	**275**
38.	How Much Does Treatment Cost?	**278**
39.	Pregnant – At Last!	**281**
40.	Preventing Infertility	**289**
41.	The Infertile Patient's Prayer and Infertility "Defined"	**294**
	Appendix 1: Semen Analysis Chart	**297**
	Appendix 2: Normal Hormone Values	**299**
	Glossary	**301**
	Index	**317**

1

How Babies are Made – The Basics

The Reproductive System of a Woman

THE SEXUAL AND REPRODUCTIVE ORGANS on the outside of a woman's body are called the *external genitals*. There are three openings in the genital area. In front is the *urethra*, from where urine comes out; below the urethra is the opening to the vagina which is called the *introitus*; and the third is the *anus* from where a bowel movement leaves the body.

The outer genital area is called the *vulva*. The vulva includes the *clitoris*, the *labia majora* and the *labia minora*. The most sensitive part of the genital area is the clitoris. This is a pea-shaped organ which is full of nerve endings and its only purpose is to provide sexual pleasure. The clitoris is protected by a hood of skin, and is the equivalent of the male's penis.

The labia majora, or outer lips, surround the opening to the vagina. They are made of fatty tissue that cushions and protects the vaginal opening. Between these outer lips are labia minora, or inner lips. These lips are sensitive to sexual stimuli. As they get stimulated, they take on a deeper colour and begin to swell.

The *vagina* is a muscular tunnel that connects the uterus (or womb) to the outside of the body. The vagina provides an exit for the menstrual fluid, and an entrance for the male's semen which is ejaculated during sexual intercourse. Normally flat, like a collapsed balloon, the vagina is extremely flexible and can stretch to accommodate a tampon, a penis or even a baby's head (during childbirth)! The walls of the vagina are muscular, smooth and soft. The vagina is a closed space which ends at the cervix.

The *uterus*, or the womb, is the place where the fertilized egg grows and develops into a baby during pregnancy. The uterus lies deep in the lower abdomen – the pelvis – and is just behind the urinary bladder. The uterus is a hollow organ shaped like a pear and is about the size of the fist. Inside the muscular walls of the uterus is a very rich lining, namely the *endometrium*, and it is in this lining that the fertilized egg gets implanted. If, however, pregnancy does not occur, this lining is shed along with blood in the form of the menstrual flow.

The neck of the uterus is called the *cervix*. It connects the uterus to the vagina and contains special glands called *crypts* that produce mucus which helps to keep bacteria out of the uterus. The cervical mucus also helps sperm in entering the uterus when the egg is ripe.

Two tubes, known as *fallopian tubes*, are attached to the upper part of the uterus on either side and are about 10 cm long. They are about as thick as a piece of spaghetti. Each tube forms a narrow passageway that opens like a funnel into the abdominal cavity, near the *ovaries* (described later). The ends of the fallopian tubes are draped over the two ovaries and they serve as a passage for the egg to travel from the ovary into the uterus. Each fallopian tube is lined by millions of tiny hairs called *cilia*, that beat rhythmically to propel the egg forward. Of course, the tube is not just a pathway – it performs other functions too, including nourishing the egg and the early embryo in its cavity. Also, the sperm fertilize the egg in one of the fallopian tubes.

HOW BABIES ARE MADE – THE BASICS

The two almond-sized *ovaries* are perched in the pelvis, one on each side, just within the fallopian tubes' grasp. The ovaries perform two functions: they produce the eggs and they also secrete hormones. Each month, at the time of ovulation, a mature egg is released by an ovary. This egg is "picked up" by the *fimbria* (a bordering fringe at the end of the fallopian tubes) and drawn into the fallopian tube.

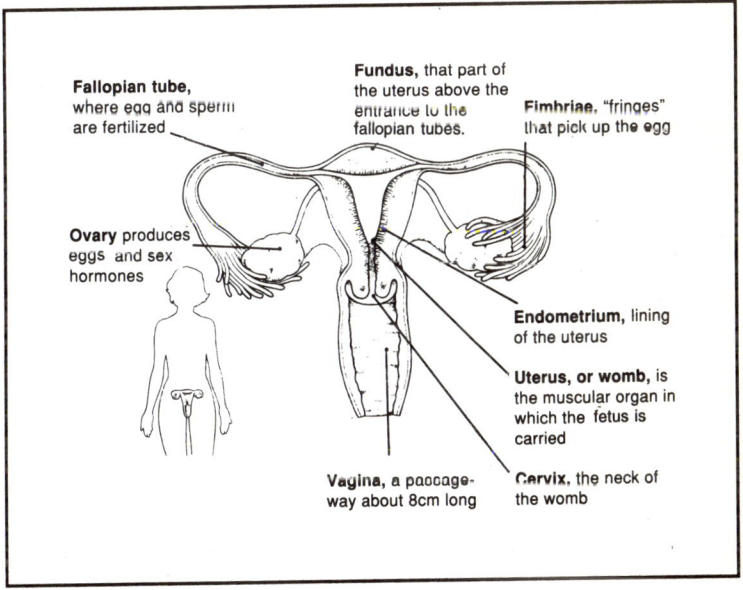

Fig. 1.1   The Female Reproductive System

How does the egg reach the fallopian tube? When ovulation occurs, the mature egg is released from the follicle in the ovary. This process of follicular rupture looks a bit like a small volcano erupting on the ovarian surface. At this time, the tubal fimbria, like tentacles, sweep over the surface of the ovary, and actually "swallow" the egg. The egg has a shell, called the *zona pellucida*, which looks somewhat like the ring around Saturn. This shell is surrounded by a cluster of nest cells called the *corona cells*, which serve to nurture the egg. These cells form the *cumulus oophorus* which is a sticky gel that protects the egg and also helps the beating of the hair-like cilia of the fallopian tube to propel the egg towards the uterus – like a conveyor belt. The egg must now wait in the protective confines of the fallopian tube, for a sperm to swim up and reach it.

The ovary contains about 2 million eggs during the sixth months of fetal life. From that point onwards, the number of eggs progressively decreases, till only about 300,000 egg cells are left at the time of birth – a lifetime's stock. During the fertile years, fewer than 500 of these eggs will be released into the fallopian tubes – once in each menstrual cycle. One of the existing eggs becomes matured for ovulation each month, and this limited supply runs out at the time of menopause. Unlike the testes in the male, which are continually churning out billions of new sperm, the ovary never produces any new eggs.

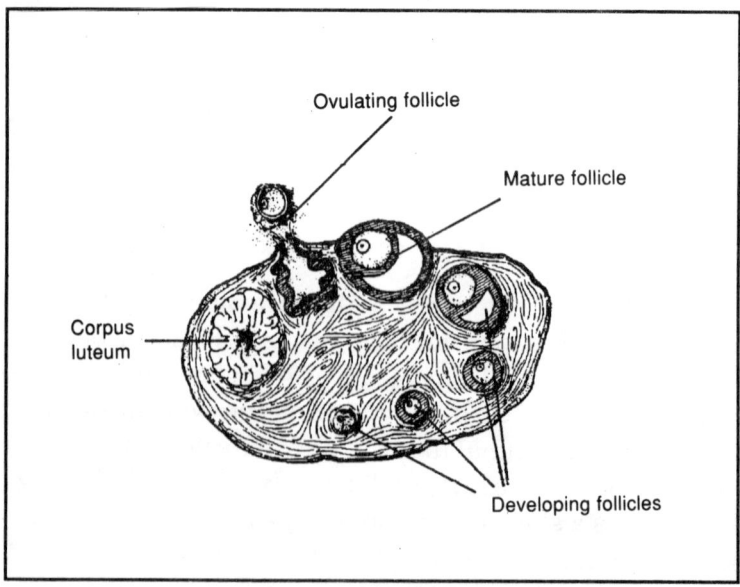

Fig. 1.2　The Ovary

The Menstrual Cycle

The aspect of the reproductive system, of which women are most aware, is the *menstrual period* or menstrual flow which they have every month. The time from the beginning of one period to the beginning of the next one is known as the *menstrual cycle*. Usually menstrual cycles last about 28-35 days, though any time period from 3 to 6 weeks is considered normal.

During the menstrual cycle, the uterus gets ready for pregnancy. Under the influence of the hormones *estrogen* and *progesterone* (see next section for details), the lining of the uterus grows rich and thick to prepare for the fertilized egg. If pregnancy does not occur, the uterus must get rid of this thick lining so that it can grow a new one in the next cycle. The old lining passes out of the uterus through the vagina as the menstrual flow.

The menstrual flow thus consists of :

(1) the shed uterine lining;
(2) blood (this comes from the blood vessels which are torn when the lining is shed); and
(3) the degenerated unfertilized egg.

If the menstrual flow is heavy, sometimes clots may be formed in it. Sometimes, the uterine lining is shed as large fragments and these fragments may sometimes look like bits of pregnancy tissue to some women, who may think they are miscarrying.

The Hormones

Reproduction is like conducting an orchestra in that the reproductive organs need to be synchronized to perform at just the right time for them to work properly and produce results effectively. It is the fertility hormones which play the conductor's role.

Hormones are chemicals that the body produces in order to carry messages from one part of the body to another. There are two major female hormones – estrogen and progesterone – which are produced by the ovaries.

The cycle of ovarian hormone production consists of two phases. In the first phase, called the *follicular phase*, estrogen plays a dominant role. During this phase the egg matures inside the ovary in its follicle, which consists of : the egg; the surrounding cells (which nurture the egg and are called *granulosa cells* and *theca cells*); and the fluid (called *follicular fluid*) which accumulates in progressively larger amounts during this phase. The follicle secretes a large amount of estrogen (produced by the granulosa cells) into the bloodstream, and this estrogen circulates to the uterus, where it stimulates the endometrium to thicken.

The second phase of hormone production begins after ovulation, midway through the cycle, when the follicle changes into a small mass of yellow tissue called the *corpus luteum*. This corpus luteum produces estrogen and also large quantities of progesterone throughout the second half of the cycle, which is called the *luteal phase* of the cycle and is named after the corpus luteum. Travelling through the bloodstream to the uterus, progesterone complements the work begun by estrogen by stimulating the endometrium to mature and making it possible for a fertilized egg to get implanted in it. In case pregnancy does not occur, the rate of production of estrogen and progesterone begins to fall 10 to 14 days after ovulation as the corpus luteum dies, and the endometrium is shed from the body during the menstrual period.

The question that arises is : How is the release of these hormones regulated by the body ? This is a complex self-regulating system, which uses negative feedback control loops, very much like a thermostat in an oven. If the temperature increases to very high levels, the thermostat shuts off the heater to reduce its heat output. When the temperature falls below the thermostat's setting, the thermostat signals the heater to turn up the heat again, thus maintaining the desired temperature. A similar signalling relationship exists between the *pituitary gland* and the ovaries (in women) and the testes (in men). The pituitary gland is a small pea-shaped structure that hangs from the base of the brain, and produces many hormones, including the *gonadotropin hormones, FSH (follicle-stimulating hormone)* and *LH (luteinizing hormone)*. As the name suggests, the function of the gonadotropin hormones is to stimulate the gonads (ovaries and testes). Thus, in the woman, FSH stimulates the growth of follicles in the ovary and the production of ostrogen; while LH stimulates production of progesterone by the corpus luteum. In the man, LH stimulates testosterone production in the testes. Production of the gonadotropin hormones by the pituitary is stimulated by the gonadotropin-releasing hormone (GnRH) secreted by the *hypothalamus*, a specialized part of the brain located just above the pituitary gland. The interplay among these hormones (GnRH; gonadotropins; and estrogen, progesterone and testosterone) regulates the reproductive system. For example, as the concentration of gonadotropins in the blood rises, this acts as a signal for the woman's ovaries to increase the hormonal output of estrogen. In turn, when the estrogen levels in the blood rise, the pituitary gland slows down its release of gonadotropins, thus maintaining the desired equilibrium.

The Reproductive System of a Man

The male reproductive system begins in the *scrotum*, which is the sack behind the penis. This sack contains two *testicles*, which manufacture a man's sex cells, called *sperm*, and the male sex hormone, called *testosterone*. The testicles feel solid, but a little spongy, like hard-boiled eggs without the shell. They hang from a cord called the *spermatic cord*.

The testicles produce sperm best when they are at a temperature which is a few degrees below the normal body temperature. This is why nature has designed a scrotum — so that the testes can hang outside the body to keep them cool.

The testicles start producing sperm when a young man reaches puberty. This is in response to the male sex hormone, testosterone, which starts being produced at this time. The testes keep on producing sperm for the rest of the man's life.

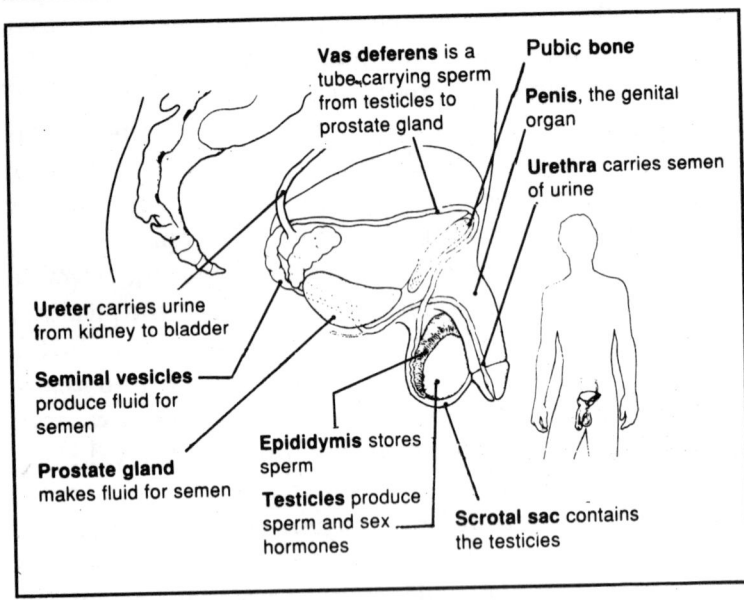

Fig. 1.3   The Male Reproductive System

The sperm are produced inside several hundred coiled microscopic tubules called *seminiferous tubules* present in the testes. These tubules converge and collect in the form of a delta (the mouth of a river) near the upper part of the testis called the *rete testis,* which then empties through a series of very small ducts, called the *efferent ducts,* out of the testis towards the *epididymis*. The epididymis is an amazing structure — it is a very long tiny tubule, which runs back and forth in convolutions and loops to form a

HOW BABIES ARE MADE – THE BASICS

tiny compact structure with a head, body and tail that sits like a cap on the top of and behind the testis. The tail of the epididymis then leads to the *vas deferens* – a thin cord-like muscular tube, which is part of the spermatic cord and which ends at the *ejaculatory duct* in the *prostate*. The prostate is a small, walnut-sized gland, which is located at the base of the bladder; and through it runs the urethra. In the prostate the ejaculatory duct is joined by the *seminal vesicle* ducts and they all open into the prostatic part of the urethra, which, in turn, leads to the urethra in the penis.

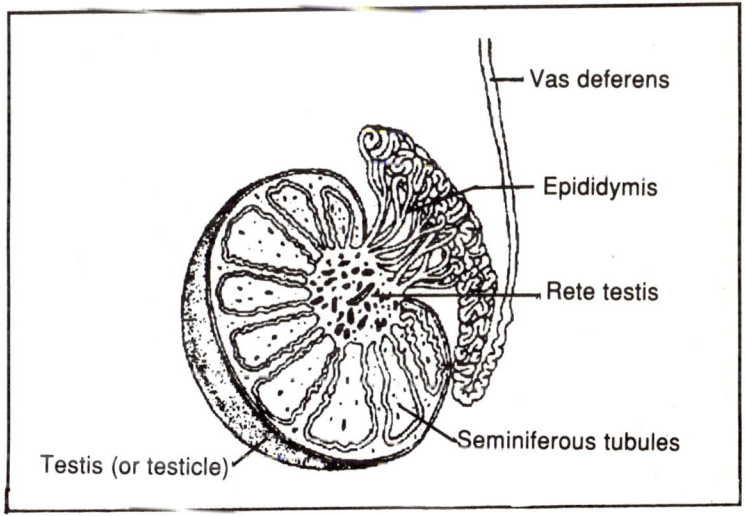

Fig. 1.4 The Testicle

Mature sperm take about 75 days to develop in a process called *spermatogenesis*. Sperm production takes place as though the sperm were on an assembly line, with the more mature sperm being passed along towards the centre of the tubule, from where they swim towards the efferent ducts of the testis towards the epididymis. This assembly line can be very "temperamental"; things may often go wrong, leading to low sperm counts.

When the sperm leave the testis, they are not yet able to swim on their own. They acquire the capacity to do so in their passage through the epididymis, which acts like a "swimming school" for the sperm. They spend between 2 and 15 days here during which they attain maturity and fertilizing potential. Sperm are propelled along this tunnel by frequent contractions of its thin muscular wall. Most of the mature sperm are then stored at the end of the epididymis, where they wait in order to be rushed through the vas deferens and then ejaculated at the time of orgasm.

During ejaculation, the muscles of the epididymis and vas deferens contract to propel the sperm into the ejaculatory duct. Here, the sperm is joined by the secretions of the seminal vesicles and the prostate gland (which contribute the bulk of the seminal fluid) to form the semen. The powerful muscles surrounding the base of the urethra then cause the semen to squirt out of the penis at the time of orgasm. The remarkable aspect of this system is that semen and urine never mix in a healthy male (even though the final passage for both is common). This is because the bladder sphincter muscle contracts during sexual stimulation, thus closing the exit from the bladder to the urethra during ejaculation, thereby preventing urine from leaking forward out of the bladder during sex and also preventing semen from accidentally going backward into the bladder.

What about the relationship between penis size and fertility ? Most men equate their fertility potential with their virility – and therefore with the size of their penis. However, the size of the penis has little to do either with fertility potential or with sexual ability. (In any case, if you worry that your penis is too small, you're not alone – most men think that their penises are too small !)

During ejaculation, about one teaspoon of semen spurts out of the penis. Semen has a milky white colour, with the consistency of egg white. Sperm account for only about 2 % to 3 % of semen. Most of the semen consists of seminal fluid, i.e., the secretion of the seminal vesicles and the prostate gland, which provide a vehicle for carrying the sperm into the vagina.

A normal ejaculation contains 200 to 500 million sperm. How can so many sperm fit into only a teaspoon of semen? Simple – sperm are very tiny. If one average ejaculation filled an Olympic size swimming pool, each sperm cell would still be smaller than a goldfish. Sperm are the smallest living cells in the human body and the egg the largest. Basically, sperm are designed so that they can deliver their contents – the male genetic material – to the egg. This is why sperm are designed like projectiles – the male DNA is found in the chromosomes in the sperm head nucleus, and the tail propels the sperm up towards the egg.

Sperm are very fragile. Consequently, very few are able to survive the hazardous swim through the female reproductive system in order to reach the egg. This is why a male produces such a large number of sperm. Perhaps the reason for this is also an "evolutionary hangover" – a legacy from our past. To amplify: female fish deposit eggs on the seabed and the male fish then sprays his sperm into the sea water. The wastage of sperm in the water is tremendous, and this is why male fish need to produce millions of sperm, in order to ensure that at least some sperm reach the eggs.

What happens to the sperm if you do not indulge in sex for many days? Unfortunately, you cannot store up sperm. If ejaculation does not occur for many days, the sperm in the reproductive ducts simply die. This is why a sperm count carried out after many days of abstinence from sex shows a high number of dead or *immotile* sperm. But there is no need to be discouraged by this. The good news is that just like you cannot store your sperm, you cannot run out of sperm either – masturbation and sexual intercourse cannot "use" sperm up. The body keeps producing sperm as long as a man has even one normal testicle.

The Role of Testosterone

As already mentioned, the main male sex hormone is testosterone and this is made by the testicles, starting at puberty. Testosterone is produced by specialized cells in the testis called the *Leydig cells*. When stimulated by the LH signal from the pituitary, these Leydig cells release testosterone into the blood stream. LH is the luteinizing hormone -- the same gonadotropin hormone found in women.

It should be noted that there are two separate compartments in the testis and that the Leydig cells are outside the spermatogenic tubules where the sperm are manufactured. This factor explains why there is no relation between virility (which depends upon testosterone production) and fertility (which depends upon sperm production).

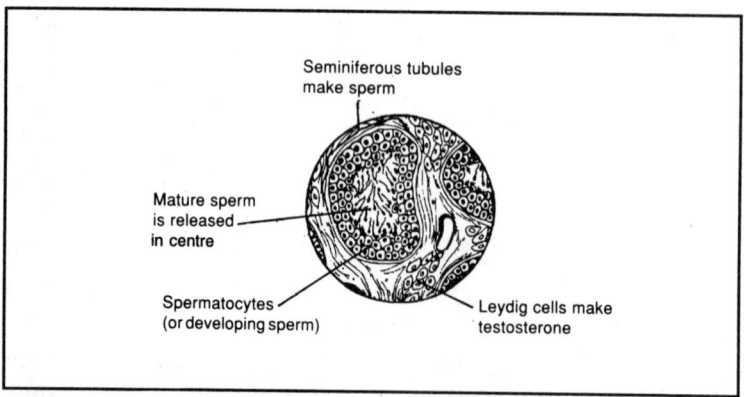

Fig. 1.5   Sperm and Hormone Production in the Testicle

Testosterone does more than just allow men to produce sperm. It also triggers the growth of facial hair, the deepening of men's voices, and the development of a male physique – all the changes which turn boys into men.

HOW BABIES ARE MADE – THE BASICS

Testosterone is also important in creating a desire for sex – it increases libido !

In addition to the need for testosterone, the production and maturation of sperm in the seminiferous tubules of the testis also require the stimulus provided by FSH produced by the pituitary gland – and this FSH is identical to that found in women.

The Sperm's Odyssey in the Female Reproductive Tract

A million million spermatozoa,
All of them alive;
Out of their cataclysm but one poor Noah
Dare hope to survive.   **Aldous Huxley**

When a man and woman have sexual intercourse, the man places his erect penis inside the woman's vagina. Here the penis releases millions of sperm when ejaculation occurs. Once the sperm have been deposited in the vagina, they have a long and arduous journey ahead of them, like salmon entering the mouth of a river to swim upstream in order to spawn. Some of the sperm swim straight up into the fallopian tubes through the cervix and uterus; and some of them swim so fast, that they have been found in the tubes in as little as a few minutes after ejaculation. Many sperm die in the acidic vaginal fluid; and some enter the alkaline cervical mucus and cervical crypts. They are stored here and can remain alive for as long as 48 to 72 hours. During this time, the sperm are released in small numbers and these continue to swim towards the fallopian tubes. (This is why you don't need to have sex every day to get pregnant, even though the egg remains alive for only 24 hours.) Sperm in the female reproductive tract swim using their own energy, generated as a result of the whip-like activity of their tail which propels them on. Of the millions of sperm released during an ejaculation, only a few hundred will survive to make the arduous trip up to the egg. Perhaps this is why so many millions of sperm are produced in the first place even though only one is needed to fertilize the egg – because the wastage is so prodigious.

The Process of Fertilization

Of the few hundred sperm which reach the egg, only one will successfully fertilize it. The process of fertilization is truly the primeval mating dance – the fertilization tango – when the female's chromosomes (in the egg) and the male's chromosomes (in the sperm) fuse together to create a new life – one which is totally different from all others, because of its unique genetic composition. As a result of advances in medical research, we have now learnt quite a lot about fertilization and this is truly one of nature's miracles.

During the time that the sperm spend in the female reproductive tract, while swimming towards the egg, they acquire the capacity to fertilize it – a process called *capacitation*. When the sperm reach the corona cells (only a few hundred successfully make the trip, guided by chemicals produced by the egg which serve as "guiding beacons" to the sperm) they become hyperactivated – they start beating their tails in a frenzy. This hyperactivation is useful because it provides the mechanical energy that the sperm head needs to burrow its way through the outer shell of the egg (called the zona). The sperm disperse the cumulus oophorus (and so far it's a team effort) and when they reach the egg, they first bind themselves to the zona. A chemical is released here by the sperm in a process called the *acrosomal reaction* in which the acrosome (which sits like a cap on the head of the sperm and behaves much like a battering ram) is removed. The acrosomal enzymes dissolve the *zona pellucida* by making a tiny hole in it, so that one sperm can swim through and reach the surface of the egg. At this time, the egg transforms the zona to an

HOW BABIES ARE MADE – THE BASICS

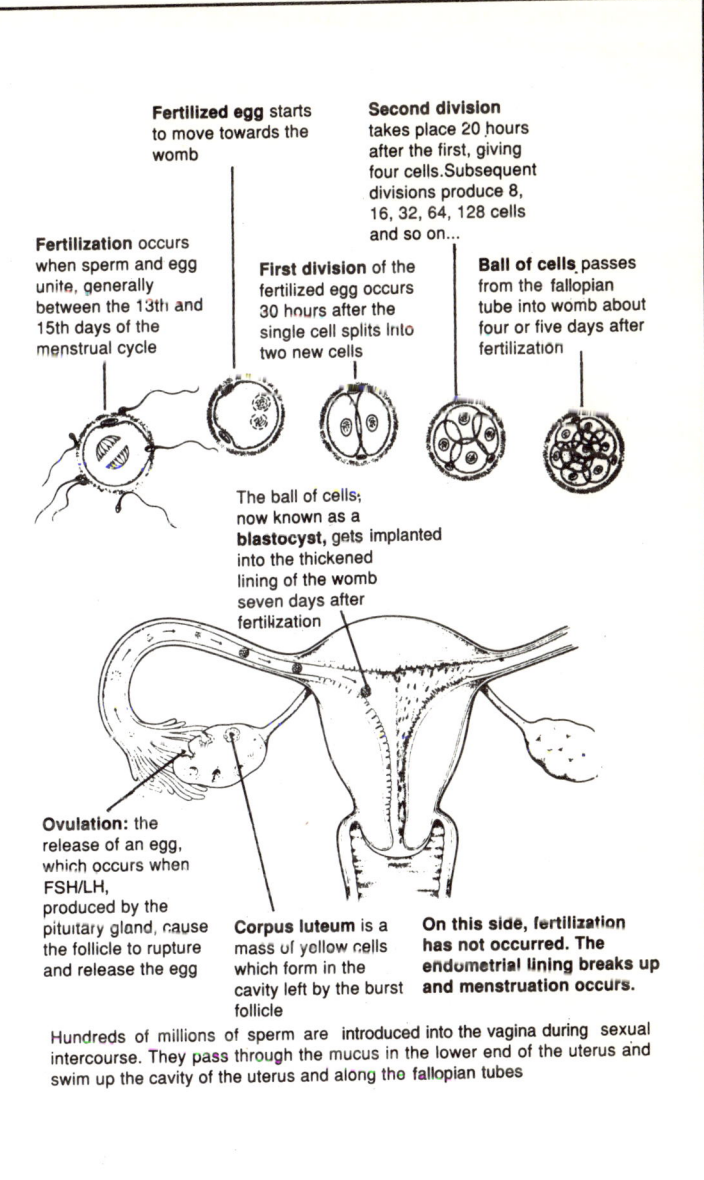

Fig. 1.6 How an Egg Is Fertilized

impenetrable barrier, thus preventing other sperm from entering.

The genetic material of the sperm (the male pronucleus) and the genetic material of the egg (the female pronucleus) then fuse — to form an *embryo*, which then divides into 2 cells. These cells, in turn, thereafter continue to divide rapidly, producing a ball of cells — now called the *blastocyst*. The embryo next travels through the fallopian tube (which nurtures it; and, at the appropriate time, propels it) into the uterus — a journey which takes about 3 to 5 days. The embryo must then break through its zona (this is called *embryo hatching*); and then attach itself to the lining of the uterus in a process called *implantation*, and, in 9 months, if all goes well, a baby will be born.

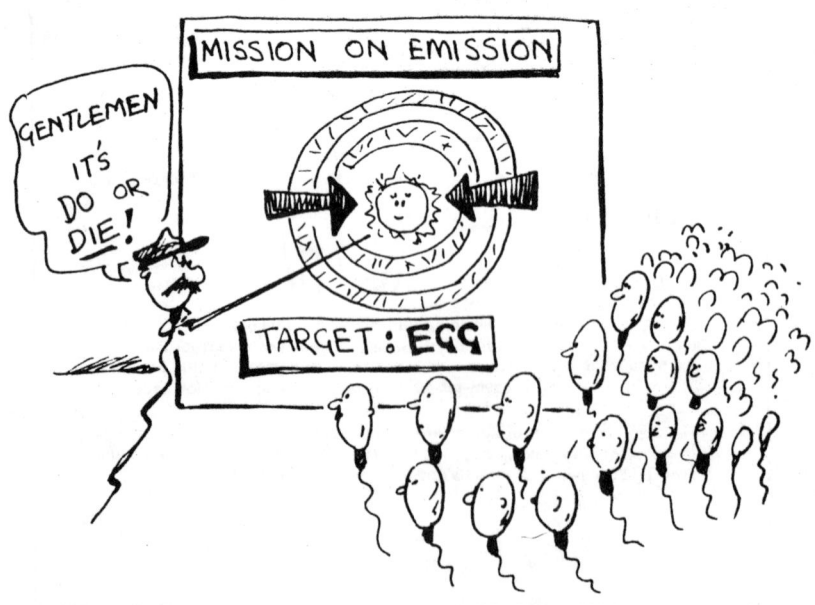

2

Do You Have an Infertility Problem? When to Start Worrying

MOST, IF NOT ALL, COUPLES EXPECT TO have their own babies once they get married. Many women naively believe that they will get pregnant the very first month they try to do so, and become concerned when a pregnancy does not occur. Most women go through a brief interlude of doubt and concern when they do not achieve pregnancy the very first month they try, and they start wondering about their fertility.

Before beginning to get worried, one should remember that, in a single menstrual cycle, the chance of a perfectly normal couple achieving a successful pregnancy is only about 25%, even if they have sex every single day. This is called their *fecundity*, which describes their fertility potential. Despite the phenomenal population growth, it should be emphasized that humans are not very efficient at producing babies! There are many reasons for this, including the fact that some eggs don't fertilize and some of the fertilized eggs don't grow well in the early developmental stage. Getting pregnant is a game of odds—it's a bit like playing Russian roulette. It's impossible to predict when an individual couple will succeed in achieving pregnancy! However, over a period of one year, the chance of achieving a successful pregnancy is between 80% and

90%; in other words, 7 out of 8 couples will be on their way to becoming parents within a year. These are the normal "fertile" couples and the rest are labelled "infertile"; the medical textbook definition of infertility being "the inability to conceive even after trying for one year". Couples who have never had a child are said to have "primary infertility"; those women who have become pregnant at least once but are unable to conceive again, are said to have "secondary infertility".

The chances of achieving pregnancy for a couple in a given cycle will depend upon many factors, and the most important ones are:

- The age of the woman. As the biological clock ticks on, the number of eggs and their quality starts decreasing.
- Frequency of intercourse. While there is no "normal" frequency for sex, the "optimal" frequency of intercourse (if the woman is trying to get pregnant) is about 3 times a week during the fertile period. Simply stated, the more sex the better! Couples who have intercourse less frequently have a diminished chance of conceiving.
- "Trying time", that is, how long the couple have been trying to get pregnant. This is an important concept. The longer a couple has been trying to conceive without success, the lesser their chances of getting pregnant without medical help.
- The presence of fertility problems.

What happens when a couple has an infertility problem? The chances of the wife getting pregnant depends upon a number of variables multiplied together. Let us consider a hypothetical example where both the husband and the wife have a condition that impairs their fertility. The husband's fertility, based on a reduced sperm count, is 50% of the normal value. His wife ovulates only in 50% of cycles;

DO YOU HAVE AN INFERTILITY PROBLEM ?

and one of her fallopian tubes is blocked. With 3 relative infertility factors, the chance of conception is calculated as follows: 0.5 (sperm count) x 0.5 (ovulation factor) x 0.5 (tubal factor) = 0.125, or 12.5% of normal. Since the chance of conception in normal fertile couples is only 25% in any one cycle, the probability of pregnancy in any given month for this couple, without treatment is only about 3% (0.125 x 25 = 0.03125)! Even if they kept on trying for 5 years, the chance of conceiving on their own would be 60% only. Thus, infertility problems multiply together and magnify the odds against a couple achieving a pregnancy. This is why it is important to correct or improve each partner's contributing infertility factors as much as possible in order to maximize the chances of conception.

If infertile couples had 300 years in which to breed, most wives would get pregnant without any treatment at all ! Of course, time is at a premium, so the odds need to be improved — and this is where medical treatment comes in.

When should you seek medical advice ?

If you have been having sexual intercourse two or three times a week at about the time of ovulation, without any form of birth control for a year or more and have not become pregnant, you meet the definition of being infertile. Pregnancy may still occur spontaneously, but from a statistical point of view, the chances are decreasing and you may now want to start thinking about seeking medical help. There is no precise "right" time to do so, and if your predicament is causing you anxiety and worry, then you should consult a doctor. Even though you may be embarrassed and feel that you are the only ones in the world facing this problem, you should not forget that you are not alone. Many couples experience infertility and many can be helped.

A note of caution should be sounded at this stage.

There are certain conditions that warrant seeing a doctor sooner:

- Periods occurring at three-week (or less) intervals.
- Periods not occurring for longer than three months.
- Irregular periods.
- A history of pelvic infection.
- Two or more miscarriages.
- Women over the age of 35 – time is now at a premium!
- Men who have had prostate infections.
- Men whose testes are not felt in the scrotum.

Tips for Self-help

Before seeking medical help, remember some of the things you can do to enhance your own fertility potential.

Body weight, diet and exercise: Proper diet and exercise are important for optimal reproductive function. Women who are significantly overweight or underweight can face difficulties in getting pregnant. Consult your doctor about a healthy diet. Normal exercise, including aerobics, tennis, or jogging, may improve your chance of conceiving. However, excessive exercise (for example, jogging over three miles per day) can adversely affect your ovulation.

Stop smoking: In men, cigarette smoking has been associated with a decreased sperm count. Women who smoke take longer to conceive.

Stop drinking alcohol: Alcohol (beer and wine as well as hard liquor) intake in men has been associated with a low sperm count.

Review your medications: A number of medications, including some of those used to treat ulcer problems and high blood pressure, can influence a man's sperm count. If you are taking any medications, have a talk with your doctor about whether or not such medication can affect your fertility.

Many medications taken during early pregnancy can affect the fetus. It is important to inform your doctor that you are attempting to become pregnant before taking prescription medications or over-the-counter medications, such as aspirin, antihistamines, or diet pills.

Stop abusing drugs: Drugs such as marijuana and anabolic steroids decrease sperm counts. If you have used drugs, discuss this aspect with your doctor. This is confidential information. Both partners should stop using any illicit drugs if they want a healthy baby. Also, limit your caffeine (tea, soft drinks and coffee) intake.

Frequency of intercourse: The simple rule is : as often as you like; the more often you have sex, the better your chances. Thus, for couples who have sex only on weekends (often the price they pay for a heavy work schedule) the chance of having sex on the fertile preovulatory day is only one-third that of couples who have sex every other day. This means they (the "weekenders") may take three times as long to conceive.

Timing of intercourse: Unlike animals, who know instinctively when to have sex in order to conceive (because the female is in "heat" or estrus when she ovulates), most couples have no idea when the woman ovulates. Timing intercourse during the "fertile period" is important and can be easily learnt . However, some couples are so anxious about having sex at exactly the right time that they may abstain for a whole week prior to the "ovulatory day" — and often the doctor is the culprit in this overrigorous scheduling of sex. Such overattention can be counterproductive (because of the anxiety and stress it generates) and is not advisable.

Position and technique of intercourse: A very interesting fact of nature is that pigs are very efficient at conserving semen — the boar literally screws his penis into the vagina of the sow, obtaining a tight lock prior to ejaculation, to ensure that no semen leaks out. Humans do not have such well-designed mechanisms of technique; perhaps this is because they are really not necessary. Most doctors advise a male superior position and also advise that the woman remain lying down for at least 5 minutes after sex and not wash or douche afterwards. A number of products used for lubrication during intercourse, such as petroleum jelly or vaginal cream, have been shown to affect sperm quality. Therefore, these products should be avoided if you are trying to get pregnant (a suitable alternative is raw egg white).

Is Fertility Lower at Present?

Has the fertility of couples declined in modern times ? Possibly. The reasons for this downfall include the following :

(1) The increasing age of women at the time of marriage and child bearing.
(2) The increased incidence of sexually transmitted diseases (STDs) which damage the reproductive tract in both men and women.
(3) Decreasing sperm counts in men which is a global phenomenon. An interesting observation made recently has been that men's sperm counts worldwide have been falling in the last few decades. Whether this phenomenon is due to environmental pollution, or due to the stresses of modern day life, remains unclear.

Where to Get Help

Most couples usually consult their family physician, who will refer them to an obstetrician-gynecologist when infertility poses problems. This first visit should include both partners. The physician will usually outline the possible causes of infertility, and provide an evaluation plan. The first step should be to achieve an accurate diagnosis to try to find out why pregnancy isn't occurring. Once a diagnosis has been determined, the couple and physician should meet again and chalk out a treatment plan. For difficult and complex problems, an infertility specialist should be consulted.

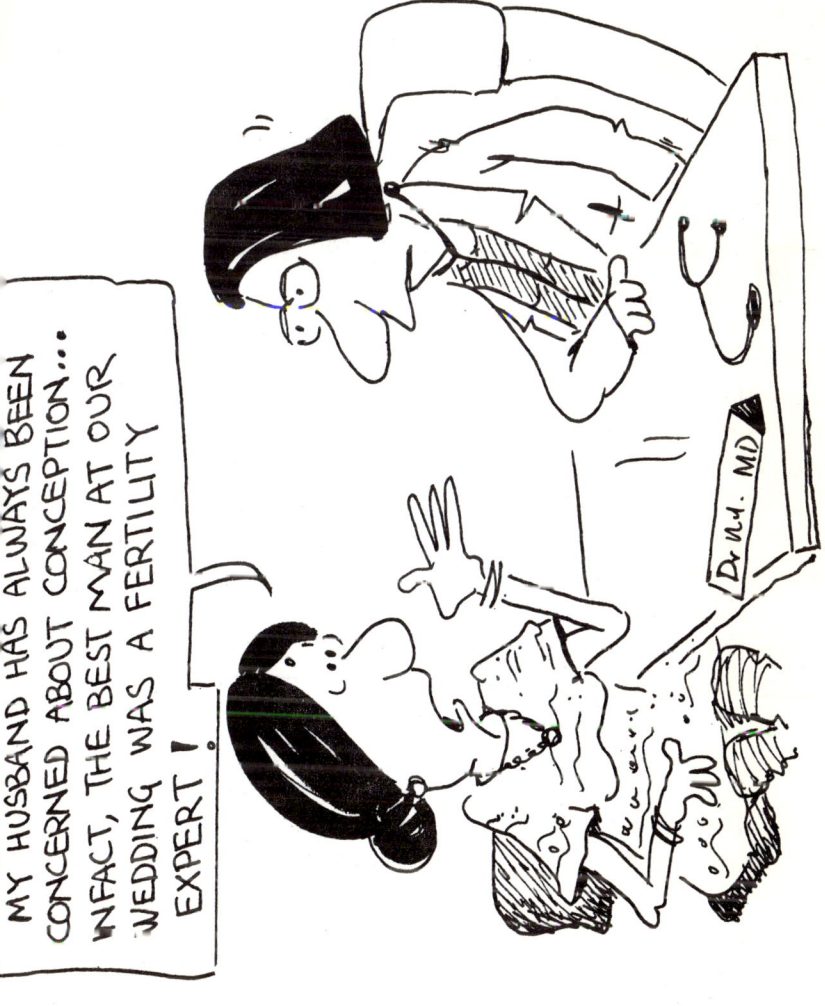

3

Finding Out What's Wrong – The Basic Medical Tests

IN ORDER TO UNDERSTAND WHY PREGNANCY doesn't occur, we need to examine the four critical areas which are needed to make a baby – eggs, fallopian tubes, sperm and embryo implantation. The required tests, which often seem endless, will actually fall into one of these areas. In 40% of the cases, the problem will be with the male, in 40% with the female, and in 10% both partners will have a problem. In some cases, about 10%, no specific cause can be identified (unexplained infertility) even after exhaustive testing.

Before starting with tests, the doctor obtains a detailed medical history from the couple, and also performs a physical examination of both of them, in order to determine if this can provide clues as to the cause of the problem.

For most couples, however, detailed investigations are needed to establish a diagnosis. The specialized tests involved in such investigations constitute the infertility workup and they can be completed efficiently in as little time as one month. Timing the procedures properly during the menstrual cycle is very important and we have found the following strategy useful in our practice.

The first day when the menstrual bleeding starts is called Day 1, and the semen analysis can be done at this

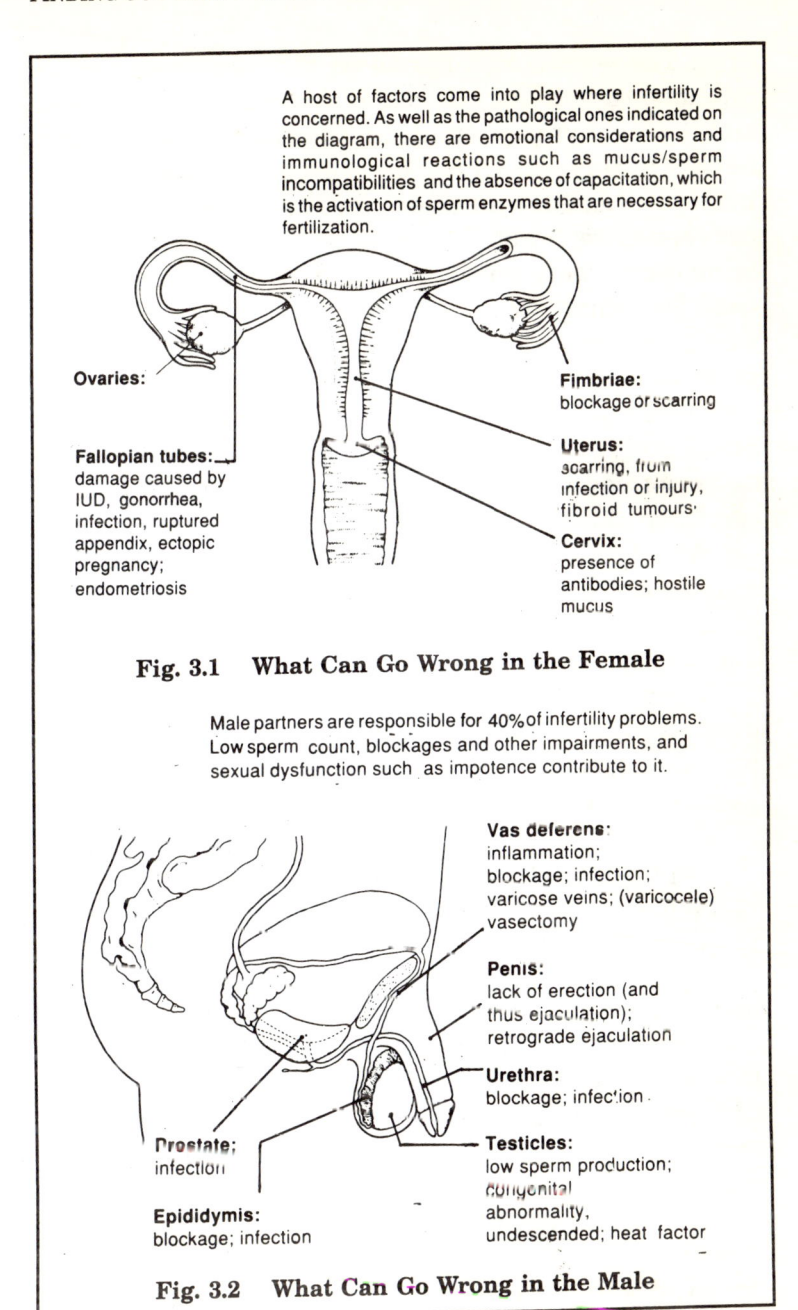

FINDING OUT WHAT'S WRONG – THE BASIC MEDICAL TESTS 25

A host of factors come into play where infertility is concerned. As well as the pathological ones indicated on the diagram, there are emotional considerations and immunological reactions such as mucus/sperm incompatibilities and the absence of capacitation, which is the activation of sperm enzymes that are necessary for fertilization.

Ovaries:

Fallopian tubes: damage caused by IUD, gonorrhea, infection, ruptured appendix, ectopic pregnancy; endometriosis

Fimbriae: blockage or scarring

Uterus: scarring, from infection or injury, fibroid tumours

Cervix: presence of antibodies; hostile mucus

Fig. 3.1 What Can Go Wrong in the Female

Male partners are responsible for 40% of infertility problems. Low sperm count, blockages and other impairments, and sexual dysfunction such as impotence contribute to it.

Vas deferens: inflammation; blockage; infection; varicose veins; (varicocele) vasectomy

Penis: lack of erection (and thus ejaculation); retrograde ejaculation

Urethra: blockage; infection

Testicles: low sperm production; congenital abnormality, undescended; heat factor

Prostate: infection

Epididymis: blockage; infection

Fig. 3.2 What Can Go Wrong in the Male

time. The wife's blood hormonal tests for prolactin, LH (luteinizing hormone), FSH (follicle-stimulating hormone) and TSH (thyroid-stimulating hormone) can be done between Days 3 and 5 of the cycle; followed by a hysterosalpingogram (X-ray of the uterus and tubes) between Days 5 and 7. Ultrasound for ovulation monitoring is done between Days 11 and 16; and the results are used for timing the PCT (postcoital test) as well, during which time the cervical mucus is also assessed. A serum progesterone level is then measured on Day 21, about 7 days after ovulation, and this level provides information about the quality of ovulation. The laparoscopy can also be performed in the same month (Days 20-25) and this can be combined with an endometrial biopsy, if desired.

With the foregoing strategy, time is not wasted, and couples can be reassured that a possible reason for the cause of the infertility, if it exists, will be detected within one month.

The workup should not stop when a single problem is discovered; it is still important to complete the testing procedures, since it is possible that infertile couples may have multiple problems.

A single test abnormality does not necessarily mean that a problem exists and the test may need to be repeated the following month, in order to confirm that the problem is a persistent one.

Unfortunately, it is very common to find that tests are done piecemeal, or sometimes, not done at all. Often, treatment is started even before establishing a diagnosis. Conversely, some doctors take so long to do the tests, that patients get fed up – after all, they don't want tests and more tests – what they want is treatment and ultimately a baby!

The doctor should meet the couple together and the first test which should be done is a semen analysis. Sadly, sometimes the wife would have undergone innumerable

FINDING OUT WHAT'S WRONG – THE BASIC MEDICAL TESTS

tests (sometimes repeatedly!) and the husband's semen analysis (where the problem lies) would not have been done even once!

It is only after the workup has been completed that a treatment plan can be formulated; and, at this stage, the couple will need to make decisions about treatment options, which are discussed in detail in subsequent chapters.

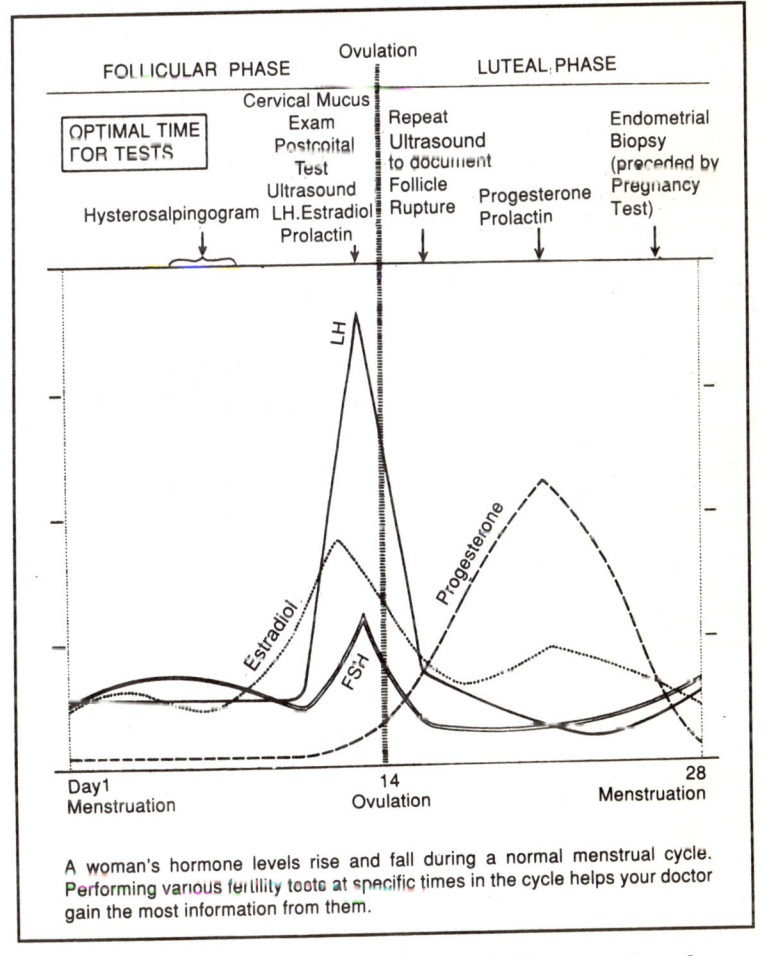

A woman's hormone levels rise and fall during a normal menstrual cycle. Performing various fertility tests at specific times in the cycle helps your doctor gain the most information from them.

Fig. 3.3 Rise and Fall of a Woman's Hormone Levels during a Normal Menstrual Cycle

4

Testing the Man : Semen Analysis

IN THE PAST, INFERTILITY WAS BLAMED wholly and solely on the woman. Perhaps this was because the male psyche equated fertility with virility and viewed failure to father a child with shame. Studies today, however, show that 40% of infertility emanates directly from the man.

The vast majority of men have simply no way of judging their fertility before getting married (unless, of course, they have indulged in a premarital affair, which has resulted in a pregnancy – the ultimate proof of male fertility!) Rarely, however, some men may know that they have a fertility problem: for example, they may suffer from a sexual problem of impotence, which prevents consummation of the marriage; or from one of hypospadias (in which the urethra is located at the base of the penis and the semen cannot be ejaculated into the vagina); or from undescended testes (in which both the testes are not in the scrotum).

When testing a couple for infertility, the man must always be tested first. Tests for the woman are far more complicated, invasive and expensive; it is much simpler to find out if the man has a problem.

The most important test is a simple and inexpensive one, namely, the semen analysis. In fact, its simplicity can be misleading, because if this test is done badly (as it often is by poorly trained technicians in small and ill-equipped laboratories), its results can be very misleading.

For a semen analysis, a fresh semen sample (not more than half-an-hour old) is needed, after sexual abstinence for at least 2 to 4 days. The man masturbates into a clean, wide mouthed bottle which is then delivered to the laboratory.

Providing a semen sample by masturbation can be very stressful for some men — especially when they know that their counts are low; or if, in the past, they have encountered problems with masturbation "on demand" for semen analysis. Men who have faced this problem can seek help. Either their wives can help them to provide a sample; or else they can see some sexually arousing pictures or use a mechanical vibrator to help them get an erection. If the problem still persists, it is possible to collect the ejaculate during sexual intercourse in a special silicone condom (which is non-toxic to the sperm but is presently not available in India), and send this condom with the ejaculate to the laboratory for testing.

The semen sample must be kept at room temperature (20°C to 30°C); and the container must be spotlessly clean. If the sample is spilt or leaks out, the test becomes invalid and needs to be repeated. Lubricants should not be used during masturbation for semen analysis as some of them can kill the sperm. It is preferable that the sample be produced in the clinic itself, and most infertility centres will have a special private room (a "masturbatorium") to allow you to do so.

How is the Test Performed in the Laboratory ?

After waiting for about 30 minutes after ejaculation, to allow the semen to liquefy, the technician or doctor will check the semen in order to determine the following factors:

The volume of the ejaculate: While a lot of infertile men feel that their discharge of semen is "too little", in reality, abnormalities of volume are not very common. They usually reflect a problem with the accessory glands – the seminal vesicles and the prostate – which produce the seminal fluid. The normal volume is about 2 ml to 6 ml. A very low volume will cause problems, because too little semen may mean that the sperm would find it difficult to reach the cervix. A very high volume of semen, surprisingly, will also cause problems, because this dilutes the total number of sperm present, thereby decreasing their concentration.

The viscosity: During ejaculation the semen spurts out as a liquid which gels promptly. This gel should liquefy again in about 30 minutes so as to allow free motility to the sperm. If the gel fails to liquefy, or if it is very thick in consistency even after liquefaction, this suggests a problem – usually one of infection of the seminal vesicles and the prostate.

The pH: Normally, semen is alkaline (pH more than 7.0). An alkaline pH protects the sperm from the acidity of the vaginal fluid. An acidic pH (less than 7.0) suggests problems with the function of the seminal vesicles.

The presence of a sugar called fructose: This sugar provides energy for sperm motility, and its absence suggests a block in the male reproductive tract.

The most important test is the examination of the semen under the microscope. What do sperm look like? Sperm are microscopic creatures which look like tiny tadpoles, swimming about at a frantic pace. Each sperm has a head, which contains the genetic material of the father, and a tail which lashes back and forth to propel the sperm along.

Request the laboratory technician to show you the sperm sample under the microscope. If normal, the sight of all those sperm swimming around can be very

reassuring. You are likely to be awestruck by the ma
numbers and the frenzy of activity. If the test is abnormal,
seeing for yourself gives you a much better idea of what
the problem is! A good laboratory should be willing to
show you the sperm sample under the microscope, and to
explain the problem, if any, to you.

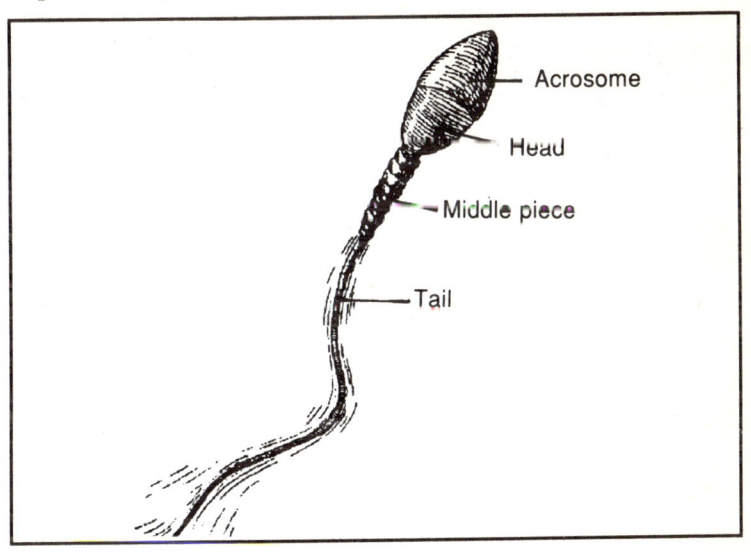

Fig. 4.1 A Normal Sperm

Under the microscope, the doctor checks to see :

If there are enough sperm. If the sample has less than 20
million sperm per ml, this is considered to be a low sperm
count, and less than 10 million is considered very low. [The
technical term for this deficiency is *oligospermia* (*oligo*
means few).] Some men have no sperm at all and are said
to be *azoospermic*. Such a result can come as a rude shock
because the semen in these patients looks absolutely
normal — it is only on microscopic examination that the
problem is detected.

Whether the sperm are moving well or not. This
movement is called *sperm motility* — and only the sperm

which move forward fast are able to swim up to the egg and fertilize it; the others are of little use. The sperm motility is graded from one to four, as follows. Grade 4 sperm are those which swim forward fast in a straight line (linear, progressive motility) like guided missiles. Grade 3 sperm swim forward, but either in a curved or a crooked line, or slowly (slow linear or non-linear motility). Grade 2 sperm move their tails, but do not move forward (non-progressive motility). Finally, Grade 1 sperm do not move at all (immotile). Sperm of Grades 2 and 1 are considered poor.

Whether the sperm are normally shaped or not – what is called sperm form or *morphology*. Ideally, a good sperm should have a reguar oval head, with a connecting midpiece and a long straight tail. If too many sperm are abnormally shaped (round heads; pin heads; very large heads; double heads; absent tails), this means that the sperm are abnormal and will not be able to fertilize the egg.

If there is sperm clumping or *agglutination*. Under the microscope, this is seen as the sperm sticking together to one another in bunches. This factor impairs sperm motility and prevents the sperm from swimming up through the cervix towards the egg.

Putting it all together, the doctor estimates the total number of good sperm in the sample – and this is calculated by multiplying the total count, the progressively motile sperm and the normally shaped sperm. This product gives the progressively motile normal sperm count which is a crude index of the fertility potential of the semen sample. Thus, for example, if a man has a total count of 40 million sperm per ml; of which 40 % are progressively motile and 60% are normally shaped, then his progressively motile normal sperm count is calculated as follows:

$$40 \times 0.40 \times 0.60 = 9.6 \text{ million progressively motile normal sperm per ml.}$$

The doctor also checks to find out whether pus cells are present or not. While the presence of a few white blood cells in the semen is normal, a large number of pus cells suggests the presence of infection in the reproductive tract.

The sperm test needs to be done meticulously. A normal sperm report is reassuring, and usually does not need to be repeated. Quite often, if the semen analysis is normal, most doctors will not even examine the male, since such examination is considered superfluous.

Poor sperm tests can result from the following factors:

- Incorrect semen collection technique, i.e., the sample is not collected properly or the container is dirty or contaminated.
- Too long a time delay between providing the sample and its testing in the laboratory.
- Too short an interval between the previous ejaculation and the test sample.
- Recent systemic illness in the last 3 months (even a flu or a fever can temporarily depress sperm counts).

If the initial sperm test proves to be abnormal, further tests will need to be repeated 3-4 times over a period of 3-6 months to confirm whether the abnormality is persistent or not. This is because sperm counts do tend to vary on their own, and it is best to repeat this test several times before coming to any conclusion. It takes six weeks for the testes to produce new sperm — which is why you need to wait before repeating the test. It also makes sense to get the repeat test done from another laboratory.

What if the sperm count is persistently poor ? Then other tests are advised, in order to try to pinpoint the problem. These tests are described in the next chapter.

5

Beyond the Semen Analysis

FOR THE MAN WITH A POOR SEMEN SAMPLE, additional tests which may be recommended include specialized sperm tests; blood tests; and testis biopsy.

Antisperm Antibodies Test

The role of antisperm antibodies in causing male infertility is controversial, since no one is sure how common or how serious this problem is. However, some men (or their wives) will possess antibodies against the sperm, which immobilize or kill them and prevent them from swimming up towards the egg. The presence of these antibodies can be tested in the blood of both partners, in the cervical mucus, and in the seminal fluid. However, there is little correlation between circulating antibodies (in the blood) and sperm-bound antibodies (in the semen). There are many methods of performing this test, which can be quite difficult to standardize, as a result of which there is a lot of variability between the result reports of different laboratories. The older methods of testing used agglutination methods on slides and in test tubes. Perhaps, the best method available today is one which uses *immunobeads*, which allow determination of the location of the antibodies on the sperm surface. If they are present on the sperm head they can interfere with the sperm's ability to penetrate the egg; if they are present on the tail they can retard sperm motility. Of course, if the test is negative, this is reassuring; the problem really arises when the test is positive! What this signifies and what to do about it are highly vexatious issues in medicine today, and doctors are even more confused about this aspect than the patients.

Semen Culture Test

In the semen culture test, the semen sample is tested for the presence of bacteria, and, if present, their sensitivity to antibiotics is determined. Interpreting this test can also be problematic ! It is normal to find some bacteria in normal semen samples — and the question which must be answered is : are these bacteria disease-causing or not ?

Tests which assess the sperm's ability "to perform" include the following sperm function tests.

Postcoital Test

The postcoital test is the easiest test of sperm function, since it is performed *in vivo*. It is done when the wife is in the "fertile" period, during which time the cervical mucus is profuse and clear. The gynecologist examines a small sample of the cervical mucus, under the microscope, a few hours after intercourse. Finding 5-10 motile sperm per high power microscopic field means that the test is normal. A normal test implies normal sperm function and can be very reassuring.

An abnormal test needs to be repeated and, if the problem is persistent, one needs to determine if the defect lies in the sperm or in the mucus, by cross-testing with the husband's sperm, donor sperm, wife's mucus and donor mucus.

Bovine Cervical Mucus Test

The bovine cervical mucus test is another form of testing for the ability of the sperm to penetrate and swim through cervical mucus, with the difference that in this case, the mucus used is that of a cow (since this is commercially available abroad in a test kit). The sperm are placed in a column of cervical mucus and how far the sperm can swim forward through the column in a given amount of time is checked with the help of a microscope.

Sperm Viability or Sperm Survival Test

This is a simple test, which provides crude (but useful!) information on the functional potential of the sperm. The sperm are washed using the same method which is used for IVF (either a Percoll spin or sperm swim up) and the washed sperm are then kept in a culture medium in the laboratory incubator for 24 hours. After 24 hours, the sperm are checked under the microscope. If the sperm are still swimming actively, this means that they have the ability to "survive" *in vitro* for this period – and this is reassuring. If, however, none of the sperm are alive after 24 hours, this suggests that they may be functionally incompetent.

Sperm Penetration Assay (SPA, Hamster Assay)

Since the basic function of a sperm is to fertilize an egg, scientists were very excited when they found that normal sperm could penetrate a denuded (zona-free) hamster egg. A zona-free hamster egg is obtained from hamsters and the covering (the zona) removed by using special chemicals. The eggs are then incubated with the sperm in an incubator in the laboratory. After 24 hours, the eggs are checked to ascertain how many sperm have been able to penetrate the egg. The result gives a penetration score, which gives an index of the sperm's fertilizing potential. This is a very delicate technique and is not available in India. In any case, nowadays scientists the world over are quite disenchanted with the test, since the correlation between IVF results (the ability to fertilize human eggs) and the SPA (the ability to penetrate zona-free hamster eggs) is quite poor.

Other specialized semen tests include:

- Testing for acrosomal status.
- HOS test – hypo-osmotic swelling test – which tests for the integrity of the sperm membrane.
- CASA – computer-assisted sperm analysis.
- Hemizona assay.
- Electron microscopy of sperm.

The aforementioned tests are highly sophisticated and are not easily available. Another drawback is that these tests are often not standardized adequately, so that interpreting their results can be quite difficult.

The ultimate sperm function test is the IVF, since this directly assesses whether or not the husband's sperm can fertilize the wife's eggs. The best way to perform this test is to culture some of the eggs with the husband's sperm and the others with donor sperm of proven fertility, at the same time. If the donor sperm can fertilize the eggs, and the husband's sperm fail to do so, then the diagnosis of sperm inability to fertilize the egg is confirmed. However, even this test is not infallible, since it has been shown that about 5% of sperm samples which fail to fertilize an egg in the first IVF attempt, can do so in a second attempt at IVF.

Blood Tests for Men

The serum FSH (follicle-stimulating hormone) level test is a very useful one for assessing testicular function. If the reason for the azoospermia or severe oligospermia is testicular failure, then this is reflected in a raised FSH level. This is because, in these patients, the testis also fails to produce a hormone called *inhibin* (which normally suppresses FSH levels to their normal range). A high FSH level is usually diagnostic of testicular failure. This test is done by a radioimmunoassay or ELISA test, and since it is a sophisticated test, it is best done in a specialized laboratory. Abnormal test results should be repeated for confirmation. The other reason for a high FSH level in some men is the consumption of *clomiphene* (a medicine often prescribed for the empiric treatment of oligospermia). This is why the test should be done only when no medication is being taken. While a high FSH level is diagnostic of testicular failure, a normal FSH level provides no useful information. A low FSH level is found in patients with hypogonadotropic hypogonadism. This is an uncommon (but treatable!) cause of azoospermia.

Along with an FSH level test, most doctors also do an LH (luteinizing hormone) level test, which provides mostly the same information.

A testosterone level test provides information on whether or not the testes are producing adequate amounts of the male hormone, namely, testosterone. Most infertile men have normal testosterone levels, because the compartment for testosterone production is separate from the compartment which produces sperm, and is usually intact in infertile men. A low testosterone level causes a decreased libido and this can be treated by testosterone replacement therapy (in the form of weekly injections or tablets). Of course, this therapy will not increase the sperm count.

In patients affected by azoospermia, there are basically only two reasons for the absence of sperm. One is because no sperm are being produced due to testicular failure. The other is that the sperm are being produced, but the outflow passage is blocked (ductal obstruction). The first test which needs to be done in these patients is an FSH level test. If this level is high, it means the problem is testicular failure and no further testing is called for. If, on the other hand, the FSH level is normal, then a testis biopsy is needed.

Testicular Biopsy

A testicular biopsy is done in order to find out whether sperm production in the testis is normal or not. This is the "gold standard" for judging testicular function, since here the testicular tissue is being examined directly.

How is a testicular biopsy performed ? This is a simple surgical procedure, which can be done under a local anesthetic, in the operating theatre or even in the doctor's clinic, if it is well equipped. The test takes about 5-10 minutes to be carried out; and a biopsy could be taken from just one testis, or from both testes, depending upon the nature of the problem.

The removed bit of tissue is then placed in a special preservative fluid, which is then sent to a pathologist for examination under a microsocope after staining.

The biopsy surgery doesn't hurt, because the local anesthetic numbs the tissues. There may be a dull ache for a few days after the procedure, but this can be relieved by mild analgesics.

Since testis biopsy is a surgical procedure, most doctors would use it as the last resort when testing the man. Often, if the FSH blood level is high (which implies testicular failure), or if the testes are clinically very small and atrophic, the doctor may decide there is no point in doing the biopsy, since it will have little impact on the treatment. If you are advised to have a testis biopsy, ask the doctor how the result will change your treatment (a question you should ask before being subjected to any medical test, in fact!).

The interpretation: While the biopsy is an easy test to perform, it is difficult to interpret properly, unless done by an expert. The doctor looks for evidence of sperm production in the seminiferous tubules. In some cases, there is no sperm production at all (absent spermatogenesis); or the sperm production is arrested at a particular stage (maturation arrest). This implies testicular failure, which is usually irreversible, and there is no treatment for this malady. If, on the other hand, sperm production in the testes is completely normal, and yet there are no sperm in the ejaculated semen, this clearly means that there is a block in the male reproductive tract. This is the one condition in which a testis biopsy is extremely useful (i.e., in the evaluation of the azoospermic male, to determine if there is a block to sperm transport).

A testis biopsy is often a procedure which is done badly because it is so minor — so beware! It is preferable that the biopsy be done by a specialist; a poorly done biopsy may make reconstructive surgery on the epididymis more difficult later on, by causing adhesions and fibrosis (scarring). The commonest problem with the biopsy, however, is that the biopsy result is not reported accurately by the pathologist. Interpreting a testis biopsy is difficult and requires special expertise — and is not something that the ordinary pathologist does well. You should retrieve and retain your own slides and preserve them carefully. The pathology laboratory can also be instructed to keep the tissue (" blocks") carefully. It is unfortunately common to find that a testis biopsy has to be repeated simply because the first one was done so badly that its results could not be accurately interpreted. It may also be a good idea to get a second specialist's opinion on the testis biopsy slides.

Vasography is another surgical test in which a radio-opaque dye is injected into the vas to determine if it is open, and, if blocked, to find out the exact site of the block. This test requires very delicate surgery and X-ray equipment and is a very infrequently done procedure because it can damage the vas.

For some men with testicular failure, a *karyotype* (study of the chromosomes) is useful, because it allows one to determine if a chromosomal problem (e.g., *Klinefelter's syndrome*, 47, XXY, with an extra X chromosome) is responsible for the azoospermia. While there is no treatment for this disorder, at least the test result provides an answer to the question of why the testes have failed -- a question which, unfortunately, medicine today still cannot answer, in the majority of patients.

6

Diagnosis and Treatment of Male Infertility – More Confusion !

THE COMMONEST REASON FOR MALE infertility is a low sperm count, and the commonest reason for this is what doctors call "idiopathic" – which simply means, we do not know! This is one of the reasons why the diagnosis of male infertility is so frustrating for both patients and doctors – there are very few tests available which allow us to pinpoint the cause of the problem. This drawback also means that there is very little in the form of effective therapy which we can offer these men; if we do not know what is wrong, how can we treat it? However, what about those conditions which we do understand? Let's now discuss these conditions in detail.

Varicocele

One of the commonest reasons for a low sperm count according to some doctors is a *varicocele*. A varicocele is a swollen varicose vein in the scrotum, usually on the left side. It usually causes no aches or pains. The condition occurs because blood gets pooled in the testicular veins (pampiniform plexus) since the valves in the veins are leaky and do not close properly. The reasons for infertility associated with a varicocele are unclear. Perhaps the accumulation of blood causes the testes to become hot and thus damage sperm production; or the pooled blood brims over with abnormal hormones which may change the way in which the testes make sperm. The effect of the varicocele on an individual's sperm count is variable; this may range from no effect whatsoever, to causing a very low sperm count. Varicoceles may also have a progressively damaging effect on sperm production, so that the sperm count may decline with time.

How is a varicocele diagnosed ? The doctor examines the patient in the erect position and feels the spermatic cord – the cord-like structure from which the testis hangs. The patient is also asked to cough at this time. A varicocele feels like a "bunch of worms" and, on coughing, this gets transiently engorged. Confirmation of this diagnosis is best done by a Doppler test at the same time. The instrument used in the Doppler test is a small pen-like ultrasound probe which is applied to the cord. This probe bounces sound waves off the blood vessels and measures the amount of blood flowing through the veins, and this can be recorded. Patients with a varicocele have a reflux of blood during coughing which shows up as a large spike on the tracing. Other somewhat uncommon tests which are done to confirm the diagnosis of a varicocele include: special X-ray studies, called venograms, and thermograms.

What are the areas of controversy regarding the varicocele? Most doctors are still not sure whether a varicocele causes a low sperm count or not ! It is possible that the varicocele may be an unrelated finding in infertile men – a "red herring". Strangely enough, only a quarter of the men with varicoceles have an infertility problem. Thus, many men with large varicoceles have excellent sperm counts which is why correlating cause (varicocele) and effect (low sperm count) is difficult.

The foregoing contention means that surgical correction of the varicocele may be of no use in improving the sperm count; after all, if the varicocele is not the cause of the problem, then how will treating it help ? Nevertheless, surgery for varicocele repair is simple and straightforward; and since there is so little we can do in any case for most men with a low sperm count, most doctors will repair any varicoceles they find in infertile men. However, it should be kept in mind that varicocele surgery will result in an improvement in sperm count and motility in only about 50% of the patients. And it is still not possible for the doctor to predict which particular patient will be benefited. Of course, merely improving the sperm count is not enough; and pregnancy rates after varicocele repair alone are around 25% only.

There are three methods available to repair varicoceles: conventional surgery; microsurgery; and radiologic balloon occlusion.

In conventional surgery, the most commonly performed procedure is as follows: a small cut is made in the groin; the spermatic cord is lifted out of the scrotum; and the engorged veins are tied off. In this case, the risks include: the risk of the varicocele recurring, which is about 20%, because some of the smaller veins are not identified and are missed out during surgery; the risk of formation of a hydrocele, i.e., a collection of fluid around the testes, because lymph vessels are indirectly tied off too, so that more fluid is accumulated (the risk is about 5%); and inadvertent damage to the testicular artery (the blood supply to the testis) -- which can actually decrease sperm production !

Microsurgery is a newer method, in which under an operating microscope, the surgeon ties off individually the enlarged veins in the spermatic cord. The testicular artery and lymphatic ducts can be preserved confidently, because the surgery is done under high magnification.

Radiologic balloon occlusion is not very commonly performed. In this rather minor procedure, a silicone balloon catheter is passed under X-ray guidance up to the testicular vein. Here, the balloon is inflated and left in place permanently, thus blocking the engorged veins and repairing the varicocele.

Subclinical varicoceles are tiny varicoceles which cannot be felt by the doctor, but can be detected by Doppler examination. Whether correcting them is helpful or not is still a matter of individual opinion.

Many surgeons will combine varicocele repair with medical therapy to try to increase the sperm count by driving the testis to work harder, but the efficacy of this method is still not clear.

Duct Blockage

If the passage (reproductive tract) between the penis and testes is blocked, there will be no sperm in the semen (azoospermia). Blockages can be caused by infection (due to gonorrhea, chlamydia, filariasis, or TB) or by surgery done earlier to repair hernias or hydroceles.

A long and complicated two- to three-hour microsurgery called a *vasoepididymal anastomosis* (VEA) can be attempted to bypass the duct blockage. This surgery requires highly specialized skills and is best performed by an experienced microsurgeon, since the tubes involved are very fine and delicate. This surgery is technically difficult and intricate because it needs to be done under high magnification. The surgeon tries to bypass the block, so that the sperm can reach the penis.

Surgical results can be poor for the following reasons:

- Technical difficulty, because of the minute size of the tubes; often, patency cannot be restored, and the sperm count remains zero. The anatomic patency rate is about 50% for most patients (which means that sperm can be found in the semen after surgery).

- The sperm are often poor in quality and are successful in giving rise to a pregnancy in only about 25% of the patients. This is because the sperm that make their way out may not be mature or motile since they have not spent enough time in the epididymis, which functions to mature the sperm in the body.
- Secondary damage to the epididymis and duct system may have occurred because they have been subjected to high pressure for a long time, causing multiple leaks and blocks, making surgery less successful.
- Damage to the functional lining of the epididymis may be present, either as a result of the infection which caused the block or as a result of the high pressure, so that it no longer works effectively and sperm cannot mature here properly.

The first surgical attempt offers the best chance of success; repeat surgery has a dismal success rate and is rarely worthwhile.

Congenital Absence of the Vas (the sperm-carrying tube)

For patients without a vas deferens (a condition they are born with, but which can be diagnosed only much later on), the conventional treatment consisted of creating a pouch surgically, into which the epididymis was made to open. This pouch was called a *spermatocele* and sperm were aspirated from it and used for artificial insemination. However, pregnancy rates were very low. Recently, a technique developed by Dr Sherman Silber of USA allows some of the men (without a vas deferens) to father a child. This technique is called MESA (microepididymal sperm aspiration), in which sperm are aspirated by microsurgery from the head of the epididymis and used for fertilizing the wife's eggs *in vitro* by IVF.

Vasectomy

Men often undergo *vasectomy* to render them sterile once they have completed their family. Vasectomy is a simple, safe and easy surgical procedure which involves cutting the vas deferens and sewing it shut, so that the sperm passage is blocked. These sperm are absorbed into the body so that although ejaculation is normal, there are no sperm present in the semen.

If the man changes his mind after a vasectomy, and wants to father another child, microsurgery can rejoin the cut ends so that the sperm can once more pass through into the semen. This reversal surgery is called *vasovasostomy* or VVA (*vasovasal anastomosis*). Such surgery is expensive and only a few doctors are adequately trained to perform the operation -- and even then success is not guaranteed. The best results are obtained in those cases where the reversal surgery has been performed within 5 years after the vasectomy, i.e., before antibodies to the sperm are developed. Competent surgeons have reported pregnancy rates of as high as 80% in these cases.

Immunity Problems with Sperm

If varicoceles are controversial, sperm immunity problems are even more so! However, while the controversy surrounding varicoceles has now become quite old, the discovery of immune sperm problems is a relatively newer development, which means we have even more questions about these problems, and even fewer answers!

In one of Nature's quirks, men can develop antibodies to their own sperm, or the wife can develop these against the husband's sperm. What actually happens is that the man's body's defence mechanism destroys its own sperm; or the wife's hostile cervical mucus does so, as though the sperm were enemy bacteria or virus. This can happen as a result of problems due to inflammation, injury to the testes, surgery, infection, or blockage.

Problems start right from making the diagnosis. Antisperm antibodies are suspected to be present when the sperm are clumped to one another (agglutinate) while doing a semen analysis. A poor postcoital test, which shows that most sperm in the cervical mucus are immotile, is also a tipoff, because one of the reasons for this finding is cervical mucus hostility due to the presence of antibodies.

Many tests are available to detect antisperm antibodies. A blood test for antisperm antibodies can be done for both the wife and the husband using ELISA methods. This is an easy test to perform but interpreting the result is difficult – what does a postive test mean? Could it be responsible for infertility? Most doctors don't think so, because they argue that the presence of these antibodies in the blood is of little clinical importance. But the debate still goes on! Antibody tests can also be done on the sperm itself, using immunobead tests, which can tell the doctor whether the antibodies are present on the sperm head or tail.

Treatment for sperm immunity problems is equally confusing, and includes administering testosterone injections to suppress sperm production; the rationale being that if there are no sperm there will be no further formation of the antagonistic antibodies.

Corticosteroids have also been used successfully to suppress the production of antibodies. But the side effects of these powerful drugs are several, and quite adverse.

Other methods such as sperm washing to clean away the seminal fluid (which contains the antibodies) along with timed insemination, and IVF (*in vitro* fertilization) and GIFT (gamete intrafallopian transfer) can also be useful.

Hormone Imbalance

Unlike in the woman, hormone imbalance in the man is not a common cause of infertility problems. Hormonal problems can stem from organs as far apart as the brain or the testicles, and can show up in blood tests. Hormone imbalance can arise because of :

- Head injury.
- A tumour in the pituitary gland, at the base of the brain.
- A tumour in the adrenal gland, above the kidneys.
- Malfunctioning of the pituitary gland.
- Cirrhosis of the liver.
- Conditions present from birth, such as Klinefelter's syndrome (47, XXY syndrome).
- A thyroid problem.

One uncommon problem is that of *hyperprolactinemia* (i.e., a high prolactin level). This problem is usually caused by a pituitary malfunction or tumour, and can be detected by a blood test. Patients with hyperprolactinemia often also have decreased libido and some may be impotent. Treatment with bromocryptine in order to suppress the high prolactin levels has proved highly successful in achieving pregnancy.

Another problem pertains to that of *hypogonadotropic hypogonadism* (poor functioning of the testes because of inadequate stimulation by the gonadotropic hormones, FSH and LH, produced by the pituitary gland). Most hypogonadotropic patients are hypogonadal; that is, their blood levels of testosterone, the male hormone, are low. This means that they have poorly developed secondary sexual characters; an effeminate appearance; scanty hair; decreased libido; and small flabby testes. Such a condition can be confirmed by blood tests which show low levels of FSH and LH. This disorder can be treated by replacement therapy with the gonadotropin hormones, i.e., HCG (human chorionic gonadotropin) and HMG (human menopausal gonadotropin). These are expensive injections and a fairly long course of treatment is needed before they begin to work, but they are effective in enhancing sperm production in these patients.

Substance Abuse

As Shakespeare once said: "Alcohol increases the desire but takes away the performance." Not only are alcoholics unable to perform, but their liver function also deteriorates, resulting in excessive levels of the female hormone, estrogen, which has a severe sperm-suppressing effect. Drugs of abuse can also create malformed sperm with poor motility; they also alter hormonal balance and testicular function and cause impotence and erection problems.

Tobacco is a potent toxin. It attacks the tails of the sperm so that they are unable to swim effectively. The testicular artery can also go into spasms if it gets choked with nicotine, and this decreased blood supply to the testis can also impair sperm production. Prolactin levels in smokers also tend to be higher, so sexual desire "disappears in smoke".

Undescended Testes

Undescended testes are a tragic cause of male infertility, since often such a condition is preventable. Some babies are born with one or both testicles up in their bellies instead of hanging down in the scrotum. Sometimes the condition might correct itself by the time the toddler is around two years old. (Don't worry unduly if you find the testes "occasionally disappearing" from the scrotum of a young boy. These testes are called "retractile" testes, and are very common.) However, if left unattended, the undescended testes tend to get damaged by the heat in the abdominal cavity and can even become cancerous in adult life. The child should be operated before two years of age or else fertility could be lost forever. Treatment with hormonal injections (HCG injections) to cause testicular descent is another alternative.

Torsion

If one of the testicles has undergone *torsion* (the doctor's term for twisting), it could be damaged since it is deprived of its blood supply.

Signs of torsion are excruciating pain and swelling of the testicles. Sadly, it is often misdiagnosed as a testis infection, and left untreated. This inaction causes the testis on that side to shrivel up and die because it gets starved of blood (a condition called *atrophy*). The best way to confirm the diagnosis of torsion of the testis is to go in for a Doppler test. If confirmed, emergency surgery is needed right away, to untwist and fix the testis properly. The other testis also must always be fixed surgically to prevent it from undergoing torsion. Unfortunately, sperm antibodies are often produced which decrease sperm production in the other testis.

Infections

Earlier, the commonest reason for azoospermia in India used to be smallpox. The smallpox virus attacked and damaged the epididymis, causing ductal obstruction. Tuberculosis also damages the epididymis, causing azoospermia. However, making a specific diagnosis of tuberculous epididymitis can be very difficult, because it is often a silent and indolent disease. Gonorrhea, chlamydia, syphilis and other STDs can also play havoc with the male genital tract, causing irreparable damage to its epithelium (internal lining).

Strange as it may seem, mumps can also cause *orchitis* (inflammation of the testes), especially when it affects young men. Orchitis can cause severe damage to the testes, resulting in testicular failure.

What about other genital tract infections? Many doctors will do a semen culture, to look for a treatable cause of infertility, if the semen sample shows many pus cells. If the test is positive treatment with antibiotics is instituted. Male reproductive tract infections (such as prostatitis) are often chronic, and may require many weeks of antibiotic treatment. It is therefore important to recheck the semen culture after therapy, to ensure that the treatment has been adequate. However, the relation between the presence of bacteria in the semen and male infertility is still unclear. Do bacteria really cause infertility? Does treating the infection help to improve fertility? More questions than answers, once again!

Medication and Its Effects

Some medications can play havoc with the sperm count or with the sex drive and these include: drugs for high blood pressure like *reserpine, methyldopa, guanethidine*, and *propranolol; nitrofurantoin* for urinary infection; corticosteroids; anabolic steroids for muscle building; and antipsychotic drugs.

A rare problem pertains to anticancer drugs and radiation therapy, which are used to treat young men suffering from cancers such as Hodgkin's disease, lymphoma, leukemia and testicular tumours. In these men, the chemotherapy and radiation therapy used to treat the disease also wipe out sperm production, rendering them sterile. An option available today is to store the sperm (in sperm banks) which can later be used for inseminating the wife to achieve a pregnancy.

Detrimental Effects of Heat

The testicles have been placed in the scrotum because they can't make sperm at body temperature – they need a cooler environment to do so. Consequently, they hang outside the body where the temperature is 0.8°C cooler. Tightly encased groins because of jock straps, tight jeans, *lungottis*, and nylon briefs cause the testicles to be pressed back into the warmth of the body and literally "cook the sperm to death" – especially when combined with hot tub baths and saunas. Heavy physical or manual labour, performed under hot conditions for long periods, like that in foundries, boiler plants and engine rooms, may also cause a lower sperm count as the testicles get too hot.

The damage due to the aforementioned factors can be prevented by wearing loose fitting cotton trousers and cotton boxer shorts, and by applying a cold towel soaked in ice water around the scrotum at least two or three times a day.

Occupational Hazards

Certain occupational hazards affect fertility by upsetting the hormonal balance, thereby suppressing sperm production.

Dangerous chemicals which have an adverse impact on fertility include the following: heavy metals, like lead, nickel and mercury; insecticides; petrochemicals; pesticides; benzene; xylene; anesthetic gases; and X- rays.

Ejaculation Problems

Very often, a perfectly fertile man may not be able to ejaculate. Since he can't make love properly he can't make babies. Some men can't even have an erection (impotence) and some cannot achieve an erection sufficient for intravaginal penetration or ejaculation in the vagina.

An older theory held that 80% of impotency problems (which are very common) were rooted in psychological inhibition and fears which could respond to sex therapy and counselling. However, modern research has lowered this figure and estimates that 50% are due to physical causes ranging from inadequate blood flow to the penis, diabetes, neurologic defects and hormonal problems.

How does the doctor suspect a physical problem? By asking a simple question: Does the individual have "wet dreams"? If men have nocturnal ejaculations (wet dreams), this would suggest that the physical apparatus is sound, and that the problem is psychological.

Testing, in this context, includes nocturnal penile tumescence (NPT) testing, which monitors for normal night-time erections, and measuring blood flow through the arteries of the penis (using Doppler methods).

The treatment that may be prescribed includes:

- Injections of papaverine and prostaglandins (chemicals which cause blood vessels to dilate) can be self-injected into the penis under medical supervision. These substances increase the blood flow to the penis, thus creating an erection.
- A surgical implant or penile prosthesis to give an artificial erection.
- Microsurgery to plug leaks in the veins of the penis, thus preventing the loss of turgidity of the erect penis.

The sperm of an individual can also be collected by masturbation and used for artificial insemination. This procedure has a very high success rate, because there is really no fertility problem as such for this patient.

Retrograde Ejaculation

Retrograde ejaculation means that the semen goes backwards into the bladder instead of coming out of the penis, so that very little or no semen is ejaculated at the time of orgasm; and the urine looks cloudy after having sex. This phenomenon occurs when the bladder sphincter muscle does not contract properly during orgasm, as a result of which the semen leaks back from the urethra into the bladder. This condition could be caused by prostate surgery, a spinal injury, diabetes, high blood pressure medication and congenital problems.

A simple way to diagnose retrograde ejaculation is to examine a man's urine after he ejaculates. If there are sperm present in the urine, this confirms the diagnosis.

DIAGNOSIS AND TREATMENT OF MALE INFERTILITY

Self-help in such a situation includes trying to have sex with a full bladder and while standing up, because this makes the muscle around the opening of the bladder more likely to stay closed. Some medications like decongestants can also help the sphincter muscle to close. Surgery can also be performed on the opening of the bladder to prevent it from misbehaving, but such a method is not very successful.

An effective treatment option is to collect the sperm and use it later for artificial insemination. After emptying the bladder, the man alkalinizes his urine by drinking soda bicarbonate and then urinates immediately after ejaculation. The sperm in the urine are recovered by special laboratory processing techniques and used for insemination. Pregnancy rates with insemination are usually low because the recovered sperm are often of poor quality and sometimes these sperm have to be used for IVF or GIFT so as to give a reasonable chance for pregnancy to occur.

Electroejaculation for Spinal Cord Problems

Men with spinal cord problems who cannot ejaculate can now father a child with the help of a new technique called *electroejaculation*. In this technique, a probe is inserted into the man's rectum and electrical stimulation is delivered to the prostate in a gradually increasing fashion to induce an ejaculation. The man usually attains an erection and ejaculates in about five minutes. The sperm recovered from this ejaculate can then be used for intrauterine insemination (IUI), IVF or GIFT, depending upon their quality (which is usually poor).

Treating the Couple

As we have seen in this chapter, if the man has a low sperm count, little can be done with conventional therapy to improve this condition. A better way is perhaps to improve the woman's fertility potential using the method of superovulation (helping her to grow many eggs). It might seem unfair that the woman is being treated for what is, essentially, the man's problem, but the fact of the matter is that there is very little effective therapy for a low sperm count and the medicines available at present are much more effective for treating the woman. Since the fertility of the couple is the sum of the fertility potential of both the partners, a male factor problem can often be treated by treating the female!

Conclusion

Conventional treatment of male infertility has poor success rates and leaves a lot to be desired. However, the availability of assisted reproductive technology in recent times has revolutionized our approach to male infertility, and using techniques such as IUI, IVF, GIFT and microinjection, many men can be helped to father their own babies. This is a rapidly developing area and spectacular advances have occurred in recent times.

7

The Case of the Man with a Low Sperm Count

MANY INFERTILE MEN ARE OBSESSED with their sperm count, and this seems to become the central concern of their lives. However, remember that the real question the man with a fertility problem is asking is *not* : What is my sperm count or motility or whatever? Rather, it is: Are my sperm capable of working or not? Can I father a baby with my sperm? Since the function of the sperm is to fertilize the egg, the only direct way of answering this question is by actually doing IVF for test fertilization. This procedure is, of course, too expensive and impractical for most people which is why other sperm function tests have been devised.

The major drawback with all these tests, however, is that they are all indirect – there is no precise correlation between test results, pregnancy rates, and fertilization *in vitro* for the *individual patient*. This is why prognosticating on abnormal sperm tests is so difficult, and why different doctors provide such widely varying interpretations based on the same sperm report.

Such a scenario is really not surprising, when you consider how abysmal our ignorance in this area is. After all, we do not even know what a "normal" sperm count is!

Since you only need one "good" sperm to fertilize an egg, we do not have a simple answer to even this very basic question! While the lower limit of the normal sperm count is considered to be 10 million progressively motile sperm per ml, remember that this is only a statistical average. For example, most doctors have had the experience of a man with a very low sperm count (as little as 2 to 5 million per ml) fathering a child on his own, with no treatment at all. In fact, when sperm counts are done for men who are undergoing a vasectomy for family planning, these men of proven fertility have sperm counts varying anywhere from 2 million to 300 million per ml. This obviously means that there is a significant variation in "fertile" sperm counts, and therefore coming to conclusions is very difficult for the doctor (leave alone the patient!).

Therefore, what is the man with a low sperm count to do? This is where we need to introduce two important concepts, namely, "trying time" and the "fertility potential of the couple". If your sperm count is low, but you have been trying to have a baby for less than one year, it still makes sense to keep on trying for about one year more, since 10% of men with low sperm counts will father a child in this time. If, however, you have already tried for more than two years with no success, you need to move on and do something more as the chances of a spontaneous pregnancy are now very low. Now, since very little can be done to improve a low sperm count (and we will come to this contentious issue later in the chapter on Understanding Your Medicines), it makes sense to try to improve the fertility potential of the woman – for example, by superovulation. If after attempting this and trying for 6 treatment cycles (the reason 6 is the magic number is that most patients who are going to become pregnant with any method will usually do so within 6 cycles) and no pregnancy ensues, you need to explore further alternatives.

What about the answer to the million dollar question: Why do I have a low sperm count? Unfortunately, nine times out of ten, the doctor will not be able to answer this question, since we do not know the answer, and no amount of testing will help us to find out. Such a condition is labelled as "idiopathic oligospermia" which is really a wastepaper basket diagnosis, and simply means "god only knows"! What we do know is that it really does not seem to be related to physique, general state of health, diet, sexual appetite or sexual frequency. While not knowing can be very frustrating, the field of medicine still has a lot to study and understand about male infertility, which is a relatively neglected field today.

The major cause of male infertility is usually a sperm problem. However, do remember that this is no reflection on your libido or sexual prowess. Sometimes, men with testicular failure find this phenomenon difficult to understand (but doctor, I have sex twice a day! How can my sperm count be low?). The reason for this is that the testis has two compartments. One compartment, the seminiferous tubules, produces sperm. The other compartment, the "interstitium" or the tissue in between the tubules (where the Leydig cells are present) produces the male sex hormone, testosterone, which causes the male sexual drive. Now, while the tubules can be easily damaged, the Leydig cells are much more resistant to damage, and will continue functioning normally in most patients with testicular failure.

Now, one can understand why the diagnosis of a low sperm count can be such a blow to one's ego — it is so totally unexpected, because it is not associated with other symptoms or signs. Different men react differently to this condition, but common feelings include: getting angry with the wife and the doctor; resentment about having to participate in infertility testing and treatment since they feel having babies is the woman's "job"; loss of self-esteem if the count remains low; and temporary sexual dysfunction such as loss of desire and poor erections.

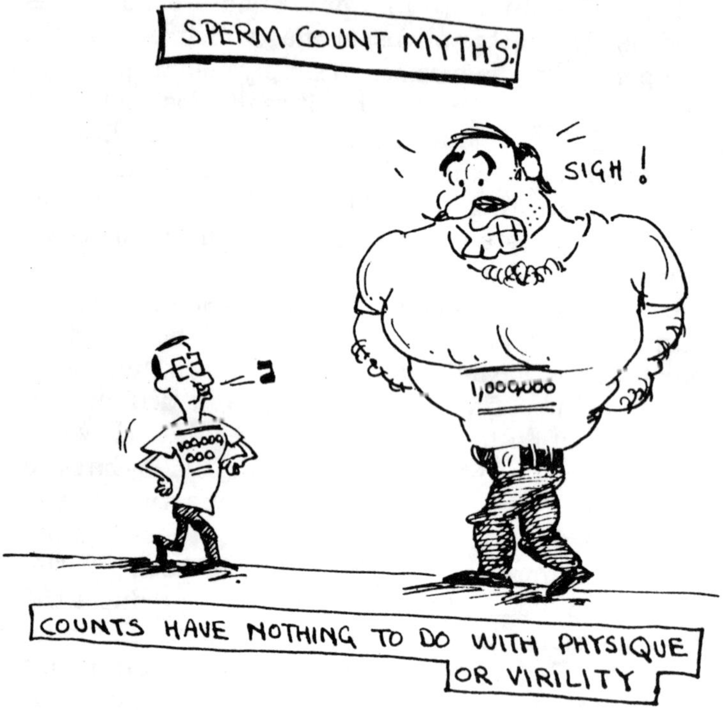
SPERM COUNT MYTHS:
SIGH !
1,000,000
COUNTS HAVE NOTHING TO DO WITH PHYSIQUE OR VIRILITY

8

Ultrasound – Seeing with Sound

ULTRASOUND OR SONOGRAPHY HAS HELPED revolutionize our approach to the treatment of the infertile patient. Ultrasound machines are the latest addition to the gynecologist's armamentarium. These machines help him to "image" or visualize structures in the female pelvis. The ultrasound technique uses high-frequency sound waves much like SONAR machines installed in ships for detecting underwater submarines. The high-frequency sound waves are bounced off the pelvic organs, and the reflected sound waves are received by a probe (called the transducer) and a computer is used to reconstruct the waves into images on the monitor. Ultrasound machines today are all real-time machines, which give dynamic images.

Earlier, ultrasound for infertility testing was done through the abdomen. Such a procedure required you to fill up your bladder (till it was ready to burst !) so that the sound waves could be transmitted into the pelvis. However, the standard ultrasound technique for infertility today is *vaginal ultrasound (endovaginal scanning)* in which a long, slim, slender probe is inserted into the vagina and used for imaging the pelvic organs. Not only is this technique much more comfortable for you but it also gives much sharper and clearer pictures, since the probe is much closer to the pelvic structures.

What can you see on ultrasound? The ultrasound gives clear pictures of the uterus and the ovaries. It allows the doctor to look for fibroids, ovarian cysts and tubal pregnancy. It is also excellent for making an early diagnosis of pregnancy. However, the ultrasound scan is not very effective for assessing whether or not the tubes are normal.

The commonest use for ultrasound today is for follicle tracking. Ovulation ultrasound scans allow the doctor to determine accurately when the egg matures and when the woman ovulates. This is often the basic procedure for most infertility treatment since the treatment revolves around the woman's ovulation. Usually, daily scans are done to visualize the growing follicle, which looks like a black bubble on the screen. Most women can see the follicle clearly for themselves, and know, by carefully looking at the scans, when the follicle has ruptured. The other useful information which can be determined by these scans is the thickness of the uterine lining – the endometrium. The ripening follicle produces increasing quantities of estrogens, which cause the endometrium to thicken. The doctor can get a good idea of how much estrogen the woman is producing (and thus the quality of the egg) based on the thickness and brightness of the endometrium on the ultrasound scan.

Who actually performs the scans? Ultrasound scans can be done either by a radiologist, or by the infertility specialist himself. The benefit of having the scans done personally by the infertility specialist is that he can make immediate decisions regarding treatment, based on the scan findings. If the radiologist does the scans, then you have to wait till your doctor has seen the report before knowing what to do next since the radiologist does not make the treatment decisions. In any case, it is preferable that the ultrasound scans be done in the infertility clinic itself, so that your waiting time can be minimized, and you don't have to run around from the sonographer to the gynecologist. If there are any abnormal findings, it is vital that your gynecologist see the actual ultrasound for himself during the scan. This provides much much more information than the printed pictures.

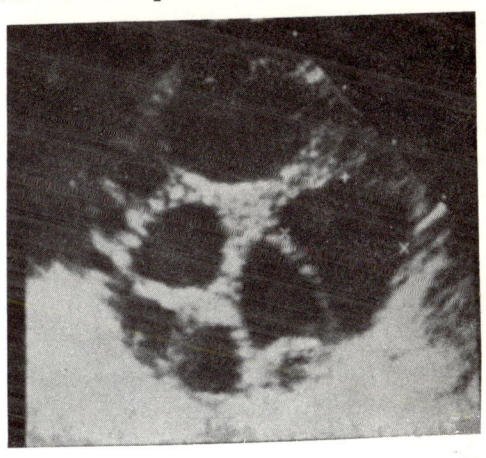

Fig. 8.1 An Ultrasound Scan of a Woman Being Superovulated. (Note the ovarian follicles which have grown; these follicles appear as black bubbles on the scan.)

Recent Advances in Ultrasound

Ultrasound technology has made dramatic advances in recent years, and now tests have been developed which allow the doctor to use ultrasound to assess patency of the fallopian tubes. Basically, these tests involve passing a fluid into the tubes through the uterus, and the gynecologist can actually see the passage of the bubbles into the tubes and out into the abdomen. Since this test (called *sonosalpingography*) can be done in the doctor's clinic itself and does not involve X-ray radiation, it offers many advantages and is especially useful for documenting that the tubes are normal. However, the present "gold standards" for tubal testing remain hysterosalpingography (HSG) and laparoscopy (described later).

The newer ultrasound machines are fitted with Doppler attachments which allow the doctor to judge the flow of blood in the blood vessels. The most exciting advance is that of colour Doppler, where the blood flow can be mapped in colour on the monitor. While still a research tool, this technique may provide important information for assessing the infertile patient in the coming years.

Ultrasound now also offers infertile patients newer treatment options not available before. Modern surgical techniques have progressively become less and less invasive – all to the patient's benefit! From laparotomy to laparoscopy, and now to ultrasound-guided procedures, we are witnessing a change in the gynecologists' armamentarium from the knife to the endoscope to the guided needle!

The advantages of the latest interventional ultrasound techniques to the patient are many and include: reduced costs; reduced period of hospitalization; reduced risk of complications; and better preservation of fertility, with increased chances of conception for the future.

Ultrasound-guided procedures can be used to treat a variety of problems encountered in infertile women.

1. *Egg pickup for IVF*: The use of vaginal ultrasound for egg pickup has made egg retrieval a short, simple and inexpensive procedure, which can be performed in a day-care unit, under sedation and local anesthesia. The ovaries are normally present in the pouch of Douglas, and are highly accessible transvaginally. Moreover, the presence of adhesions does not interfere with egg collection.

2. *Ovarian cyst aspiration*: An ovarian cyst is a very common occurrence in which fluid collects in the ovary. However, cysts which are more than 5 cm in size need to be treated, as they can cause problems (e.g., twisting and rupture). Earlier, surgery had to be done to remove these cysts, and often such surgery damaged the surrounding normal ovary as well. At present, with ultrasound guidance, the doctor can stick a needle from the vagina into the cyst, and empty the contents (usually clear fluid)

ULTRASOUND – SEEING WITH SOUND

by sucking them out. This method empties the cyst, which often does not recur.

3. *Treatment of ectopic pregnancy*: With technological advances (ultrasound and beta-HCG blood tests) the diagnosis of tubal pregnancy can be made very early, usually before the growing tubal pregnancy causes the tube to rupture. Today, under ultrasound guidance, the tubal pregnancy can be treated by injecting a toxic chemical, methotrexate, into the sac of the tubal pregnancy, which causes the tissue to die and then get reabsorbed, without any surgery whatsoever. In more advanced tubal pregnancies, potassium chloride can be injected directly into the heart of the fetus in the ectopic gestational sac, thus killing it and preventing it from growing.

4. *Ultrasound-guided tubal embryo and gamete transfer for IVF and GIFT techniques*: Techniques have been devised to pass a special catheter – the Jansen-Anderson catheter set – into the fallopian tube through the vagina under ultrasound guidance, so as to place the embryos and/or the gametes in the fallopian tube. Since the fallopian tube offers a better environment for the gametes and embryos than the uterine cavity, it is believed that this procedure will improve pregnancy rates.

5. *Tubal recanalization for cornual blocks* (proximal tubal obstruction): Often, cornual blocks occur due to the presence of mucus plugs and amorphous debris in the tubal lumen. Ultrasound-guided tubal catheterization can effectively open up the blocked tubes in some of these patients.

The scope of ultrasound-guided procedures for treating infertility has increased dramatically in the last few years; and with further improvements in this technology, we can expect the benefits resulting from ultrasound to become even greater as doctors become more versatile in using this technology.

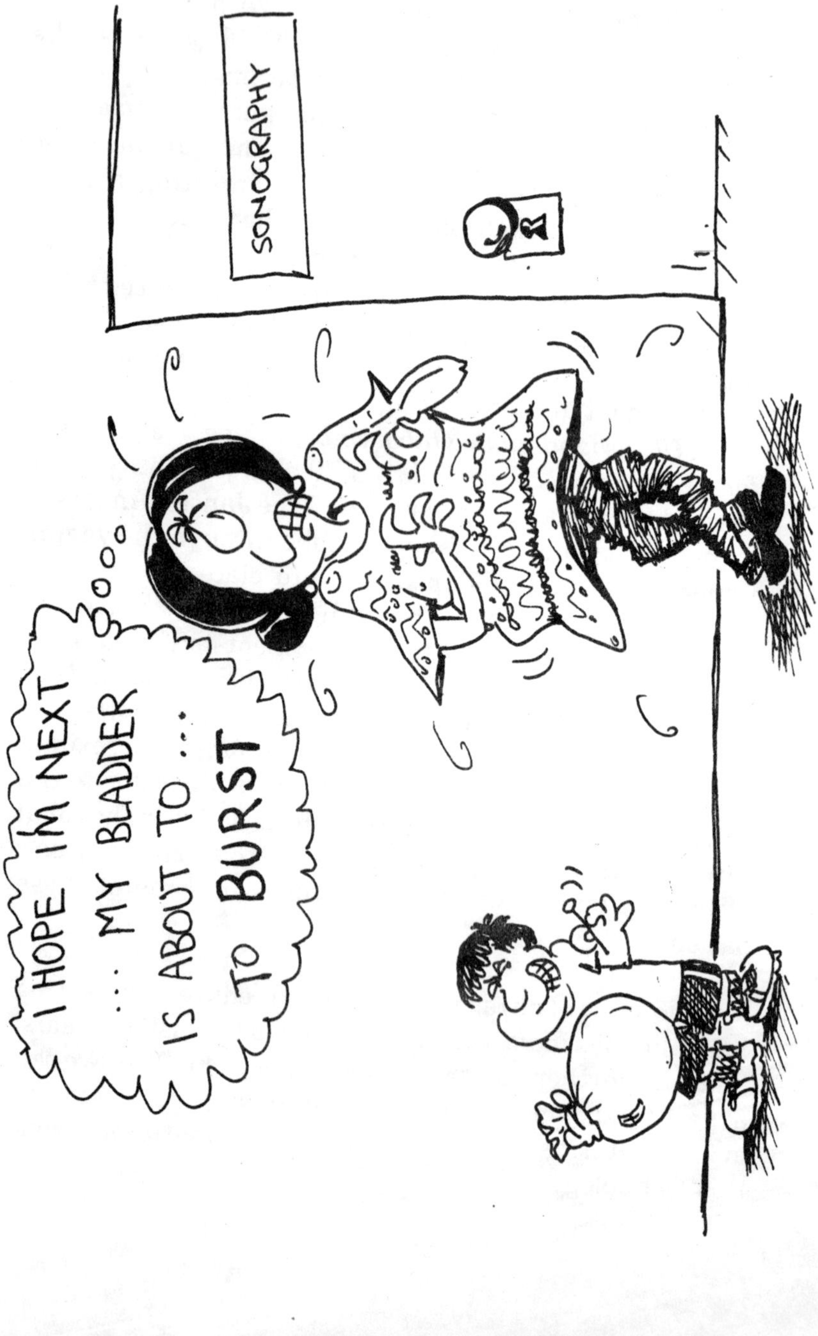
SONOGRAPHY
I HOPE I'M NEXT ... MY BLADDER IS ABOUT TO ... TO BURST

9

Laparoscopy – The Kinder Cut

LAPAROSCOPY IS A SURGICAL PROCEDURE in which a telescope is inserted inside the abdomen through a small cut below the navel, so that the doctor can have a look at the pelvic organs in the infertile woman. A laparoscopy can lead to the diagnosis of many problems which cause infertility including damaged tubes, endometriosis, adhesions and tuberculosis.

When Is Laparoscopy Done?

Most infertile women require diagnostic laparoscopy in order to complete their evaluation. Generally, the procedure is performed after the basic infertility tests, although the presence of pain or other problems (such as a history of previous surgery) may signal that a laparoscopy needs to be done before the other infertility-testing methods are performed. Most doctors will defer a laparoscopy until the rest of your evaluation is completed, since it is a surgical procedure.

Timing the Surgery

Some doctors will time the laparoscopy during the premenstrual phase (the week before the next period is due). They combine the laparoscopy with a dilatation and curettage (D & C) (scraping the inside of the uterine cavity) so that they can also get information on the woman's ovulatory status in the same procedure.

Some doctors try to perform the diagnostic laparoscopy during the periovulatory period (i.e., when the eggs are ripe, as judged by ultrasound) because such timing allows them to visualize follicular development. Some others prefer this timing so that they can treat the infertility at the same time by doing an intratubal insemination (also called SIFT or *sperm intrafallopian transfer*) in that cycle, if appropriate. This would be possible only if a previously done HSG showed that the tubes were normal.

Precautions Before Surgery

The patient is advised not to eat or drink anything for a specific time before the operation. Some tests may also be done before the procedure, to ensure safety for anesthesia, though for most young healthy women tests are usually not needed. Some doctors may want a HSG (hysterosalpingogram) done before performing a laparoscopy.

The surgery is usually done on a day-care basis. Laparoscopy is done under general anesthesia so that the patient remains asleep during surgery and does not feel any discomfort.

The Laparoscopic Procedure

First of all, the abdomen is cleansed and draped for the procedure. Then an instrument may be placed in the uterus through the vagina. A gas, such as carbon dioxide or nitrous oxide or air is then allowed to flow into the abdomen through a special needle inserted into the abdomen just below the belly button. This gas creates a space inside by pushing the abdominal wall and the bowel away from the organs in the pelvic area and makes it easier to see the reproductive organs clearly.

The laparoscope, which is a slender tube, like a miniature telescope, is then inserted through a small incision just below the navel. During the laparoscopy a small probe is placed through another incision in order to move the pelvic organs into clear view. A diagnostic laparoscopy is incomplete without a "second puncture" because, without this second probe, it is not possible to visualize all the structures completely. During the

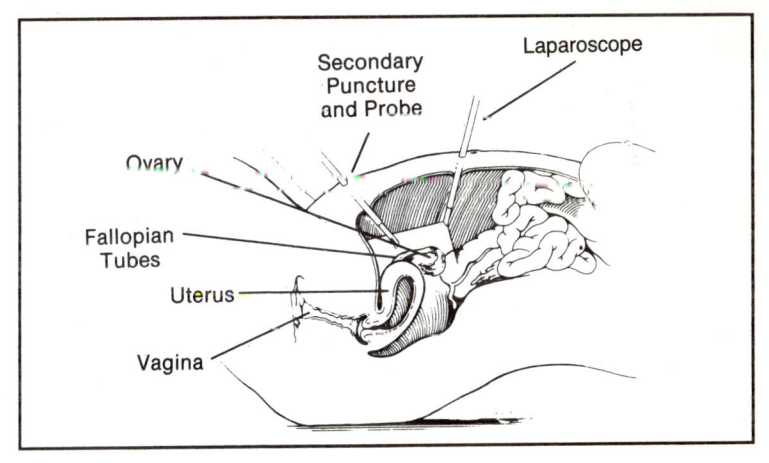

Fig. 9.1 Laparoscopy Allows the Surgeon to See the Outside of the Uterus, Fallopian Tubes and Ovaries

laparoscopy the entire pelvis is carefully scanned and the organs inspected systematically – the uterus; the fallopian tubes throughout their entire length; the ovaries; and the lining of the abdomen, called the *peritoneum*. In addition to looking for diseases affecting these structures, the doctor also looks for adhesions (bands of scar tissue), endometriosis and tubercles. In case abnormalities are found, the doctor can either try to correct them (operative laparoscopy), or take out bits of tissue for histologic examination (biopsy) with a biopsy forceps. A blue dye (methylene blue) is then injected through the uterus and fallopian tubes to check whether the tubes are open. When the surgery is complete, the gas is removed and one or two stitches inserted to close the incisions. Since the incisions are so small, often stitches are not needed and they can be closed with Bandaids.

As stated earlier, along with laparoscopy, some doctors carry out a dilatation and curettage (D & C) and send the endometrial curettings for histologic examination to rule out the possibility of hidden tuberculosis, and also to find out if ovulation is taking place. Others will do a diagnostic hysteroscopy at the same time, to ensure that the uterine cavity is normal.

Another advanced technique available now is called *videolaparoscopy*. It is possible to connect a video camera to the laparoscope, so that what the surgeon sees can be displayed on a TV monitor. This kind of laparoscopy can be very useful for documentation and record-keeping. It is also very helpful for patient education, since the doctor can use the video later on to explain to the patient the exact nature of her problem.

Operative Laparoscopy

During operative laparoscopy, many problems which cause infertility can be safely treated through the laparoscope at the same time that the diagnosis is made. When performing operative laparoscopy, additional instruments such as probes, scissors, biopsy forceps, coagulators and suture materials are placed into the abdomen, either through the laparoscope or through two or three additional incisions called "suprapubic punctures", which are made above the pubis.

Some of the disorders that can be corrected with the help of the aforementioned procedure include: releasing scar tissue and/or adhesions from around the fallopian tubes and ovaries; opening blocked tubes; and removing ovarian cysts. Endometriosis can also be destroyed by burning it from the back of the uterus, ovaries, or peritoneum during operative laparoscopy. Under certain circumstances, small fibroid tumours can be removed and ectopic pregnancies can be treated.

When performing operative laparoscopy, surgeons may use electrocautery instruments, lasers, and sutures. The choice of the technique used depends on many factors including the surgeon's training, location of the problem, and availability of equipment.

Sometimes, a "second-look" laparoscopy may be recommended. This procedure is performed following either operative laparoscopy or major tubal surgery. Second-look laparoscopy can take place within a few days following the initial surgery or many months afterwards. During the procedure, the doctor determines whether adhesions are re-forming or if endometriosis is returning and these conditions can be treated if needed.

After surgery, the patient needs to rest for about 2 to 4 hours in order to recover from the effects of anesthesia. She can usually go home the same day and resume normal work in 2 to 3 days. Sexual activity can be resumed in a week or so, depending upon the doctor's advice.

After the operation, there may be some discomfort. This may include:

- Mild nausea as a result of the medication or the surgical procedure.
- Pain in the neck and shoulder due to the gas inside the abdomen.
- Pain in the areas where the instruments passed through the abdominal wall.
- A scratchy throat and hoarse voice if a breathing tube was used during general anesthesia.
- Cramps, like menstrual cramps.
- Discharge like a menstrual flow for a day or two.
- Muscle aches.

Most of these minor symptoms will disappear within a day or two after surgery. The abdomen may feel swollen for a few days. Any unusual or peculiar symptoms should be reported at once to the doctor.

To really appreciate the benefits of laparoscopy, one should remember that the alternative is major surgery (laparotomy) which involves a large abdominal incision, a four- to six-day hospital stay, and four to six weeks of postoperative recovery time.

While the doctor may term laparoscopy as being "minor" surgery, remember that for the patient all surgery is major! The risks of laparoscopy are minimal. But certain conditions increase the possibility of complications. If there has been previous surgery in the abdomen, especially involving the bowel, there is an increased risk. Other conditions that lead to a higher risk of complications are evidence of an infection in the abdomen, a large growth or tumour within the abdomen, and obesity.

Complications among young, healthy women undergoing laparoscopy are rare and occur only in about three out of 1000 cases. These complications can include injuries to structures in the abdomen such as the bowel, a blood vessel or the bladder. Most often, these injuries occur when the laparoscope is placed through the navel. If such an injury occurs during the procedure, the physician can perform major surgery and correct the damage through a longer abdominal incision. Sometimes, complications may arise after surgery. If bleeding or pain appears excessive or if a high fever develops, the doctor should be informed.

Comparing Laparoscopy and HSG

A common question patients ask is if they can go in for an X-ray (hysterosalpingogram) instead of a laparoscopy to find out if their tubes are open? While it is true that an HSG will provide accurate information about whether or not the tubes are open, there are other major benefits which laparoscopy offers and which HSG does not. HSG provides information only about the inside of the tubes and uterine cavity, whereas in laparoscopy, not only can the tubal patency be determined, but other disorders inside

LAPAROSCOPY – THE KINDER CUT

the abdomen which affect tubal function and which do not show up on HSG (such as endometriosis and tubal adhesions) can also be diagnosed. Moreover, a major bonus in the case of laparoscopy is that it offers the doctor a chance to diagnose and treat the problem at the same time if possible – a double bonus! Of course, the advantage of HSG is that no surgery, hospitalization or anesthesia is needed; it is less expensive; and that a hard copy record is provided, which all doctors can refer to later on. In fact, both the HSG and laparoscopy are complementary procedures, and you may even need both, especially if your tubes are blocked.

A common problem which patients face in practice is that many doctors will insist on repeating the laparoscopy. One reason for this is that doctors feel that they need to do the laparoscopy for themselves, because they cannot "trust" another doctor's judgement. This is, of course, a major problem for patients, who suffer repeated (and unnecessary) laparoscopies. Having a video record should help to minimize this problem. What happens if your laparoscopy was normal and the second doctor wants to repeat it anyway? Sometimes, doctors have little to offer in the way of effective treatment and since there is nothing else to do, they suggest a repeat scopy to which the hapless patient is forced to agree. If your first scopy did, in fact, indicate you had a problem, a second look laparoscopy may be indicated (and this should have been discussed with you after the first scopy) to determine if the problem has been successfully resolved. Ask the doctor what information he hopes to get by doing the repeat laparoscopy and how this will change your treatment. If you feel the doctor wants to do a scopy for no very good reason, refuse! It's a surgical procedure after all – and it's your body!

Thinking it Over...

A major benefit of laparoscopy is that in addition to allowing the accurate diagnosis of a problem, if it exists, operative laparoscopy can also be done in the same surgery to correct the problem. Often, the laparoscopy provides reassurance that the woman is normal and that the chances of having a baby are therefore good. In such cases, it even allows the doctor to perform treatment for the infertility in that cycle, if appropriate, by using intratubal insemination or SIFT.

Laparoscopy often leads to an accurate diagnosis which, in turn, leads to more appropriate and specific treatment. Once the laparoscopy is over, the doctor will usually have a good idea of what is wrong, and what can be done about it. Whatever the problem is, the chances of it being treated effectively are improved now that the diagnosis is accurate.

After the Laparoscopy

At the follow-up visit, discuss with the doctor what he found at the time of the laparoscopy and also how to proceed on the basis of the findings. There are three possible courses of action:

1. *Normal findings* : Such findings are the commonest result and can be very reassuring !
2. *Abnormal findings*, which could be corrected at the time of laparoscopy itself : Perhaps the doctor may suggest a second-look laparoscopy or HSG after some time to document that the problem has, in fact, been corrected; or else, in addition, medical treatment may be advised, to try to correct a residual problem (e.g., antibiotics for pelvic infection; medical treatment for endometriosis). A quandary may arise when the laparoscopy reveals a finding which may be of no relevance to the problem of infertility. For example, during laparoscopy the doctor may detect small fibroids, early endometriosis, or an ovarian cyst. These are common disorders and are often found in fertile

women as well. Just making a diagnosis of these disorders does not automatically mean that they need to be corrected; they may be red herrings, which do not affect fertility. In fact, unnecessary surgery to remove these disorders can aggravate your infertility!

3. *Abnormal findings*, which could not be corrected during the laparoscopy: For treatment, the doctor may advise formal surgery (for example, microsurgery for blocked tubes) or IVF (for example, for patients with pelvic TB).

10

Hysteroscopy

HYSTEROSCOPY, AS THE NAME SUGGESTS (*hystero* = uterus; *scopy* = to see), is a surgical procedure in which a telescope is inserted inside the uterus to examine the uterine lining. This procedure can assist in the diagnosis of abnormal uterine conditions such as

1. submucous (internal) fibroids,
2. scarring (adhesions or synechiae),
3. polyps, and
4. uterine septa and other congenital malformations.

Therefore, hysteroscopy is an important tool in the study of infertility.

Before performing hysteroscopy, a hysterosalpingogram (an X-ray of the uterus and fallopian tubes) may be carried out to provide additional information about the uterine cavity, which can be useful during surgery. Diagnostic hysteroscopy is usually conducted on a day-care basis with either general or local anesthesia being administered, and takes about 30 minutes to perform.

The first step of hysteroscopy involves cervical dilatation, i.e., stretching and opening the canal of the cervix with a series of dilators. Once the dilatation of the cervix is complete, the hysteroscope, a narrow, lighted telescope, is passed through the cervix and into the lower end of the uterus. A clear solution (Hyskon or glycine) or carbon dioxide gas is then injected into the uterus through the instrument. This solution or gas expands the uterine cavity, clears blood and mucus away, and enables the doctor to directly view the internal structure of the uterus.

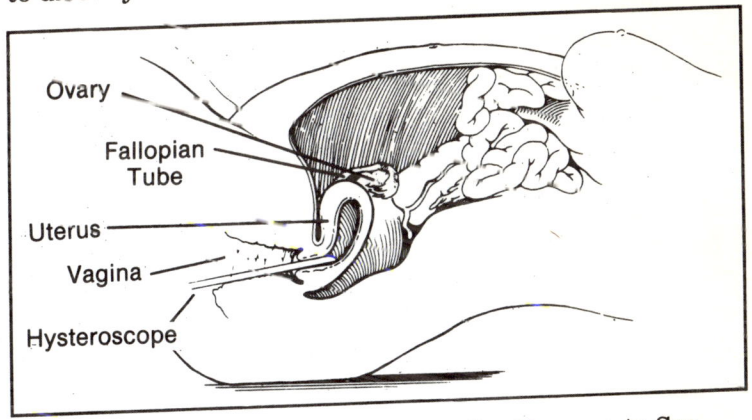

Fig. 10.1 Hysteroscopy Enables the Surgeon to See the Inside of the Uterus

The doctor systematically examines the lining of the cervical canal and the lining of the uterine cavity and looks for the internal openings of the fallopian tubes where they enter the uterine cavity – the tubal ostia.

Some doctors may do a curettage (a scraping of the inside of the uterine cavity) after the hysteroscopy and send the endometrial tissue for pathological examination.

Operative Hysteroscopy

The technique of hysteroscopy has also been expanded to include operative hysteroscopy. Operative hysteroscopy can treat many of the abnormalities found during diagnostic hysteroscopy.

The procedure in operative hysteroscopy is very similar to diagnostic hysteroscopy except that operating instruments such as scissors, biopsy forceps, electrocautery instruments and graspers can be placed into the uterine cavity through a channel in the operative hysteroscope. Fibroid tumours, scar tissue (synechiae or adhesions) and polyps can be removed from inside the uterus. Congenital abnormalities, such as a uterine septum, may also be corrected through the hysteroscope.

A very exciting new method for treating proximal tubal obstruction (cornual blocks, where the tubes are blocked at the uterotubal junction) is that of *hysteroscopic tubal cannulation*. Many studies have shown that this kind of block is often because of mucus plugs or debris which obstruct the tubal lining at the uterotubal junction which is as thin as a hair. It is now possible to pass a fine guide-wire through the hysteroscope into the tubes, and thus remove the plug or debris and open the tubes, thereby restoring normal tubal patency with "minimally invasive surgery"!

Another related advance has been the development of the method of *falloposcopy*, in which a very fine flexible telescope is passed into the fallopian tube through the hysteroscope, so as to visualize the interior of the entire fallopian tube.

After undergoing a hysteroscopy, patients often develop cramps similar to that experienced during a menstrual period and also experience some vaginal staining for several days. Regular activities can be resumed within one or two days after surgery. Sexual intercourse should be avoided for a few days (or for as long as bleeding occurs).

Complications rarely occur during hysteroscopy. In a few cases, infection of the uterus or fallopian tubes can result. Occasionally, a hole may be made through the wall of the uterus, i.e., a perforation. However, this is usually not a serious problem because the perforation closes on its own. Frequently, when extensive operative hysteroscopy is planned, diagnostic laparoscopy is performed at the same time so as to allow the surgeon to see the outside as well as the inside of the uterus to try to reduce the risk of accidental uterine perforation. Other possible complications include allergic reactions and bleeding.

Hysteroscopy, hysterosalpingography and vaginal ultrasound are all complementary procedures for evaluating the uterine cavity in the infertile woman. The HSG is useful in looking for polyps, adhesions and septa which appear as "filling defects" on the X-ray. However, a careful radiological technique is a must. Vaginal ultrasound is excellent for detecting submucosal fibroids, which can be missed during hysteroscopy and HSG. Of course, the major advantage of hysteroscopy is that it offers the chance of treating the problem as well.

11

The Tubal Connection

THE FALLOPIAN TUBES, WHICH PLAY a vital role in conception, project out from either side of the body of the uterus and form the passages through which the egg is conducted from the ovary into the uterus. The fallopian tubes are about 10 cm long and the outer end of each tube is funnel shaped, ending in long fringes called *fimbriae*. These fimbriae catch the mature egg and channel it down into the fallopian tube when it is released from the ovary. The tube itself is a highly movable muscular structure capable of precisely coordinated movement. The egg and sperm meet in the outer half of the fallopian tube, called the *ampulla*. Fertilization occurs here, after which the fertilized egg, now called an embryo, continues its way down the tube towards the uterus. The uterine end of the fallopian tube, called the *isthmus*, acts like a sphincter, and prevents the embryo from being released into the uterus until just the right time for implantation, which is about 4 to 7 days after ovulation. The tube is much more complex than a simple pipe, and the lining of the tube is folded and lined with microscopic hair-like projections called *cilia*, whose beating pushes the egg and embryo along the tube. The tubal lining also produces a fluid that nourishes the egg and embryo during its sojourn in the tube.

Tubal Diseases

Tubal abnormalities account for between 25% and 50% of female infertility. Tubal damage usually occurs through pelvic infection, often due to unknown causes. However, some of the causes of pelvic infection that can be pinpointed are :

- Sexually transmitted diseases (e.g., gonorrhea, chlamydia).
- Infection after child birth, miscarriage, medical termination of pregnancy (MTP) or IUD (intra-uterine device) insertion.
- Postoperative pelvic infection (e.g., surgery for perforated appendix, ovarian cysts).
- Severe endometriosis.
- Tuberculosis.

Besides causing blocked tubes, any pelvic inflammatory disease can also produce bands of scar tissue, called adhesions, which can alter the functioning of the fallopian tubes.

Pelvic tuberculosis is a fairly common cause of tubal damage in India. It is a silent disease, and most women suffering from pelvic tuberculosis are unaware of this fact. The tuberculosis bacteria reach the tubes from the lungs through the bloodstream and can cause irreparable tubal damage.

Making a Diagnosis of Tubal Diseases

A number of tests are available to judge whether or not the fallopian tubes are open.

The simplest and the oldest test for tubal patency is the *RT* or Rubin's test (named after its inventor). In this test, gas is passed under pressure into the tubes through the cervix and the uterus – either using a special machine (Rubin's apparatus) or with an ordinary syringe. The doctor then listens with a stethoscope placed on the abdomen to determine if he can hear the sound of gas passing through the fallopian tube. Even though this test is now obsolete, because it is so unreliable, a number of doctors still conduct it.

Hysterosalpingogram (uterotubogram) or HSG is a specialized X-ray of the uterus and fallopian tubes. An HSG is done after the menstrual flow has just stopped, usually on day 6 or day 7 of the period, at which time the lining of the uterus is thin. It is normally done in an X-ray clinic. Many doctors advise the patient to take an antibiotic and a pain-killer before the procedure. After positioning the patient on the X-ray table, the doctor places a special instrument in the cervix, called a *cervical cannula*. This instrument can be made of metal but the newer disposable ones are made of plastic. A radio-opaque dye (a liquid which is opaque to X-rays) is then injected into the uterine cavity. This is done slowly under pressure, and preferably with continuous monitoring using an image intensifier. The passage of the dye into the uterine cavity and then into the tubes and from there into the abdomen can be seen and X-ray pictures taken. These X-rays provide a permanent record.

At least three films need to be taken to provide a reliable record, including an early film for studying the uterine cavity and a delayed film to make sure that the spill in the abdomen is free.

An HSG defines the inside of the reproductive tract. In a normal HSG, this tract appears as a triangle (usually white on a black background) which represents the uterine cavity and, from here, the dye enters the tubes which appear as two long thin lines, one on either side of the cavity. When the dye spills into the abdomen from a patent (open) tube, this appears as a smudge in the X-rays.

The commonest problems on HSG appear in the tubes. If the tubes are blocked at the cornual end (at the uterotubal junction), then no dye enters the tubes and they

THE TUBAL CONNECTION

cannot be seen at all. If the block is at the fimbrial end, then the tubes get filled up but the dye does not spill out into the abdominal cavity and the end of the tubes are often swollen up. Occasionally, the HSG may also reveal a problem in the uterine cavity, such as a polyp, fibroid, adhesion or septum, and this appears as a gap or filling defect.

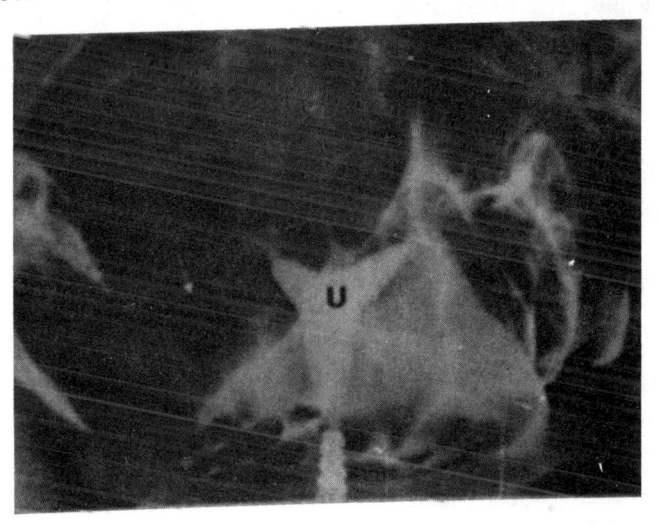

Fig. 11.1 A Hysterosalpingogram (X-ray of the Uterus). [The fallopian tubes are clearly delineated by the dye. They are seen as two long, thin lines, leading away from the triangular uterine cavity and they are clearly open (patent).]

Sometimes, like any other medical test, the HSG may provide erroneous results. For example, the cornu of the uterus may go into a spasm, as a result of which the dye may not enter the tubes at all. Such an occurrence may be interpreted as a tubal block, whereas, in reality, the tubes are open. In some women, the tubes are blocked at the fimbrial end and this is called a hydrosalpinx. However, if the wall of the hydrosalpinx is very thin and if the dye is injected under pressure, the dye may spill into the abdomen through a tear in the wall of the hydrosalpinx, suggesting tubal patency when really the tubes are closed.

While the HSG is usually very reliable for determining whether or not the tubes are open, it provides little information on structures outside the tube which could, nevertheless, impair tubal function, such as peritubal adhesions. If the spill is "loculated" (i.e., it collects in small puddles), the presence of adhesions can be suspected, but not confirmed.

An HSG can be painful and when the dye is injected into the uterine cavity, most women will experience a considerable amount of pain. You should be prepared for this and taking a pain-killer prior to the procedure will help to reduce the pain.

The doctor may encounter technical difficulties when doing the HSG for some women (especially if the cervix is too small or too tight); and it is preferable to have a gynecologist present at the time of the HSG to assist the radiologist. Many gynecologists will carry out the HSG themselves.

The major risk involved in an HSG is that of spreading an unrecognized infection from the cervix up into the tubes. Such a possibility is uncommon, but in order to reduce the risk, many doctors advise antibiotic coverage during the procedure.

If the first HSG shows that the tubes are blocked, then it may be advisable to repeat the HSG, and also to perform a laparoscopy to confirm this diagnosis.

Limitations of HSG and Laparoscopy

The trouble with both HSG and laparoscopy is that they only provide information as to whether or not the tube is open. While a closed tube will never work, they do not provide any information on how well an apparently open tube works. Remember that just because a tube is patent (open) does not necessarily mean that it works!

THE TUBAL CONNECTION

Another limitation is that both these tests will rarely provide any information as to why the tubes are blocked. Occasionally, however, the reasons can be inferred by other signs (for example, by seeing the tubercles diagnostic of TB in the abdomen during laparoscopy).

Recent Innovations in the Field

Fluoroscopic guided procedures: Using an image intensifier, and techniques borrowed from coronary angioplasty, the radiologist can now insert special catheters under fluoroscopic (X-ray) guidance into each of the fallopian tubes. This procedure is called *selective salpingography* and allows much better visualization of each tube. It also allows the radiologist to treat some cornual blocks (those which occur due to mucus plugs) by tubal cannulation.

Sonosalpingography : Under ultrasound guidance, with Doppler facilities (if available), the gynecologist can inject fluid into the tubes through the cervix and observe the flow of the fluid into the tubes and abdomen on the ultrasound screen. This is a simple bedside test which a gynecologist can perform to judge if the tubes are normal, and can be reassuring if positive.

Tuboscopy: At the time of laparoscopy, the doctor can insert a fine telescope into the fallopian tube through its fimbrial end, in order to inspect the inner lining of the tube (to judge whether or not it is healthy).

Falloposcopy: This is a very recent exciting advance, pioneered by Dr John Kerin of Australia. In this method, a very fine flexible fibreoptic tube is guided through the cervix and uterus into each fallopian tube, thus allowing the doctor to actually visualize the inner lining of the entire length of the fallopian tube – something which was never possible so far. This technique can provide useful information about the extent of tubal damage and the possibility for successful repair.

Surgical Treatment

Once the doctor has assessed the damage and pinpointed the location of the blockages he will decide on treatment alternatives and how to proceed. The first choice would usually be an attempt at surgery to repair the tubal damage. However, tubal surgery is not advisable for patients if the tubes are blocked because of TB; if the tubes are very badly damaged; or if the tubes are blocked at multiple places, because the chance for success with surgical repair for these patients is very poor. These patients may be referred directly for IVF (*in vitro* fertilization).

The likelihood of surgical success (in terms of pregnancy occurring) depends on the severity of the tubal damage. If a previous infectious process has caused scarring of the fallopian tube, the inner delicate lining may have become irreversibly damaged. Operations can result in re-establishing patency in some cases, but the main aim of the surgery is not to just open the tubes but also to achieve pregnancy. Consequently, the tubes have to become capable of capturing the egg and transporting it to the uterus for this to happen. Unfortunately, surgery cannot reverse damage to the tubal lining once this has occurred.

What if only one tube is blocked? The answer is that one normal tube is sufficient to achieve a pregnancy and most surgeons would not advise tubal surgery for these patients. Obviously, the chance of pregnancy for such patients is half that of normal women and therefore establishing a pregnancy may take them twice as long.

Tubal Microsurgery

Microsurgery entails the use of the following surgical techniques:

- Using a microscope (for adequate magnification).
- Avoiding unnecessary trauma to the tissues.

- Employing delicate surgical instruments.
- Employing fine suture (stitching) material and ensuring precise suturing.
- Handling tissues with great care and respect, to minimize tissue damage.
- Ensuring that no bleeding is left unattended and no clots are left behind (because this can lead to the formation of adhesions or scar tissue after the surgery).

The microsurgery operation may take from 1 to 4 hours, depending on the extent of pelvic damage and is usually done under spinal or general anesthesia. The incision used is usually a "bikini cut"(Pfannensteil incision). The length of stay in hospital is usually 3 to 7 days. Tubal microsurgery can be expensive and may cost up to Rs 15, 000. Sometimes a "check or second-look laparoscopy" is performed about one week after surgery to ensure that tubal patency is maintained and to remove any small adhesions that may have started to re-form.

Proximal Tubal Damage

If the tubal obstruction is at the uterotubal junction, this is called a "cornual block". The conventional surgical repair of cornual blocks involved reimplanting the tube into the uterus (and had dismal success rates). However, with microsurgery, it is possible to observe the very fine ends of the tubes under high magnification and to join them together. This technique can result in a pregnancy in about 50% of patients, since the function of the rest of the tube is basically intact.

Recently, doctors have realized that a number of patients have cornual blocks because of the presence of mucus plugs and debris in the very fine cornual segment of the tubes. Newer non-surgical methods have now been devised to treat this disorder. One of these methods involves the passage of a fine guide-wire or a fine balloon into the cornual end of the tube through the uterus, in order to dislodge the debris, and thus open the tube. This method is called a "balloon tuboplasty" or "cornual recanalization", and can be done under ultrasound guidance, hysteroscopic guidance or fluoroscopic (X-ray) guidance. This advance is a significant one, since it saves patients the need for major surgery and also achieves excellent pregnancy rates.

Salpingolysis

Salpingolysis entails the division of adhesions surrounding the tubes. When no other damage is apparent, success rates may be as high as 65%.

Tubal Reanastomosis

This technique includes a variety of procedures which involve removing the damaged portion of the tubes and rejoining the healthy ends of the tubes together. Success rates vary according to the area of damage but are usually within the range of 20-50%. The chances of success are higher when the defect occurs in the middle section of the tube.

Distal Tubal Damage

If the tubes have been severely damaged and have formed a hydrosalpinx (in which the fimbriae stick to one another and the tube is closed off), the surgery required is called *neosalpingostomy*, in which the surgeon opens the hydrosalpinx and creates a new opening for the repaired tube. While this procedure is technically easy, success rates are very poor (about 20%) because the physiologic functioning of the fimbriae rarely returns to normal.

If the damage is less severe (fimbrial agglutination, in which the fimbriae are stuck to one another; or phimosis, in which the tube is narrowed, but open), then surgical repair is more successful, with pregnancy rates being about 50%.

The risk of having an ectopic (tubal) pregnancy is increased following tubal surgery. Fallopian tubes which have been operated on may have a damaged inner lining, and this can impair the movement of the embryo down the tube. This is why, in patients who have had tubal surgery, the diagnosis of a pregnancy should be made as soon as possible (preferably within a few days of missing a menstrual period), to rule out the possibility of an ectopic pregnancy.

The best chance of success is with the first surgical operation; therefore, you need to go to a specialized centre. The chances of success will depend upon the extent of tubal damage and also on the skill of the surgeon. The best chance of achieving a pregnancy is in the first few months after surgery, and most women who are going to get pregnant after tubal surgery will conceive within this time. Some doctors believe that using ovulation induction and/or intrauterine insemination after tubal surgery helps to maximize the chances of a pregnancy.

If the patient has not conceived within one year after the surgery, then follow-up testing in the form of an HSG and/or laparoscopy is advisable, to determine whether the fallopian tubes are still open.

If the first surgery has been unsuccessful, the chance of success as a result of reoperation is very low, and such patients may be advised to try IVF.

In the future, it is possible that tubal transplants may become a reality and that scientists may also develop artificial synthetic tubes to replace damaged ones.

Operative laparoscopy for tubal repair: With recent advances in laparoscopy, it is now possible to open damaged tubes through the laparoscope, thus saving the patient major surgery. A hydrosalpinx can be repaired by opening it with a laser or cautery and then keeping it open with sutures; and even the complicated operation of tubal reanastomosis has been performed by experienced surgeons through the laparoscope (using sutures or special adhesive glue).

Reversal of Sterilization

In women, sterilization for family planning is usually done through an operation called *tubal ligation*, which is usually carried out through the laparoscope. The aim of the operation is to block the tubes and prevent the sperm and egg from meeting each other.

Why Do Women Ask for Reversal ?

The vast majority of people are very happy with sterilization. Nevertheless, there are a few women who are very distressed afterwards and would do almost anything to get things undone. The commonest reason why such women regret sterilization is because their child dies or because they have remarried and wish to bear their new husband's child.

What Can Be Done ?

If there is a reasonable amount of tube remaining, even if only on one side, then it may be possible to perform tubal microsurgery to rejoin the tubes. On the whole, the more tube which has been left undamaged, the better the chances of success. Thus, patients who have had a tubal ligation done through the laparoscope, using Falope rings (silastic bands) or clips, have an excellent chance of achieving a pregnancy after microsurgical reversal of the ligation, because these methods cause minimal tubal damage.

After reviewing the operative notes, a laparoscopy may be advised, so that the exact state of the fallopian tubes can be assessed. If the patient has enough normal tube, tubal microsurgery may be attempted and pregnancy rates can be as high as 75% in favourable cases. If, unfortunately, the patient has had both tubes completely removed or if the tubes are very badly damaged, then the only chance of success will be with IVF.

12

Ovulation – Normal and Abnormal

Normal Ovulation

NORMALLY, ONE OF THE OVARIES RELEASES a single mature egg every month. Women may experience pain or abdominal discomfort at the time of ovulation and occasionally have some slight vaginal bleeding. The presence of regular periods, premenstrual tension and dysmenorrhoea (period pains) usually indicate that the menstrual cycles are ovulatory.

Eggs are stored in the ovaries in a very immature form. In this state they are not capable of being fertilized by a sperm until they undergo a maturing process which culminates in their release from the ovary at the time of ovulation. Egg maturation and ovulation are stimulated by two hormones secreted by the pituitary, namely, the follicle-stimulating hormone (FSH) and luteinizing hormone (LH). These two hormones must be produced in appropriate amounts throughout the monthly cycle for normal ovulation to occur.

After ovulation has occurred, the follicle from which the egg has been released forms a cystic structure called the *corpus luteum*. This structure is responsible for producing progesterone in the second half of the cycle.

Most women who have regular periods have ovulatory cycles. Women who fail to ovulate or whose ovulation is abnormal usually have a disturbance in their menstrual pattern. This disturbance may take the form of complete lack of periods (amenorrhoea), irregular or delayed periods (oligomenorrhoea) or occasionally a shortened cycle due to a defect in the second part (luteal phase) of the cycle.

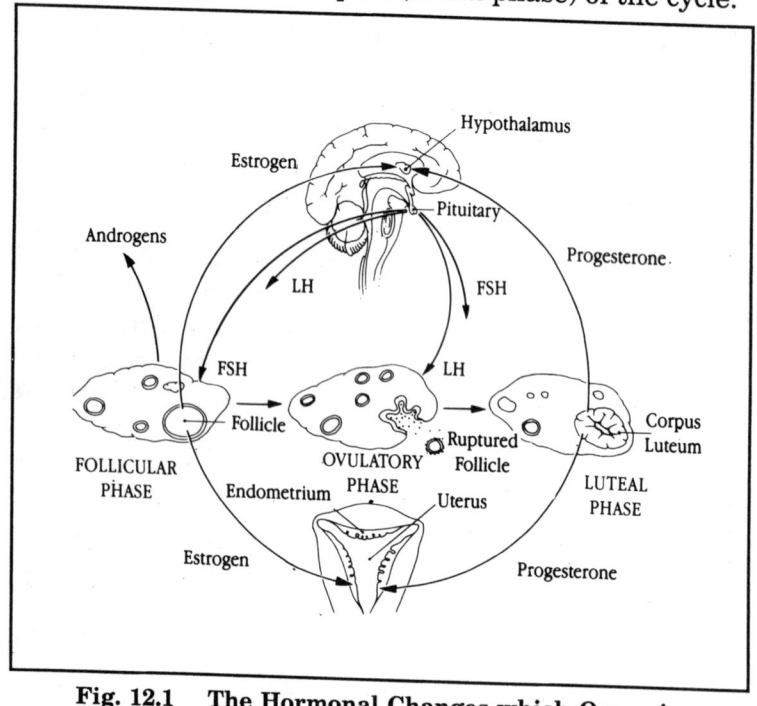

Fig. 12.1   The Hormonal Changes which Occur in a Normal Ovulatory Cycle

Detecting Ovulation

Menstrual Period Timing

To determine the length of the menstrual cycle, one only needs to note the date of the beginning of the menstrual period (first day of flow) for two consecutive periods, and then count the day from one date to the next. Keeping track of the length of menstrual cycles will help determine the approximate time of ovulation, because the next period begins approximately two weeks from the date of ovulation.

The rough rule to calculate the approximate date of ovulation is: NMP minus 14 days, where NMP is the (expected) date of the next menstrual period. This formula is based on the fact that the luteal phase for most women is constant and is 14 days' long.

Keeping track of the menstrual cycle by charting it can indicate other ovulatory disturbances. For example, if a menstrual cycle that is normally 28 days starts to occur every 35 or 40 days, this may mean that ovulation is disturbed, and that a medical evaluation is needed.

Basal Body Temperature (BBT) Chart

During the luteal phase of the cycle, the corpus luteum produces the hormone progesterone, which elevates the basal body temperature. When this temperature has gone up for several days, one can assume that ovulation has occurred. However, it is important to remember that the BBT chart cannot predict ovulation – it cannot tell you when exactly it is going to occur!

The basal temperature chart can be a useful tool. It allows the patient to determine for herself if she is ovulating as well as the approximate date of ovulation, in retrospect. Basal body temperature charts are easy to obtain and the only equipment required is a special BBT thermometer.

General instructions for keeping a basal body temperature chart include the following:

1. The chart starts on the first day of menstrual flow. Enter the date.
2. Each morning, immediately after awakening, and before getting out of bed or doing anything else, place the thermometer under the tongue for at least two minutes. This must be done every morning, except during the period.

3. Accurately record the temperature reading on the graph by placing a dot in the proper location. Indicate days of intercourse with a cross.
4. Note down any obvious reason for temperature variation such as colds, or fever on the graph above the reading for that day.

The major limitation of the BBT chart is that it does not tell you in advance when you are going to ovulate; therefore its utility in timing sex during the fertile period is small. Interpreting the BBT charts can be tricky for many patients – rarely do the charts look like those you see in textbooks! Also, keeping a BBT chart can be very stressful– taking your temperature as the first thing you do when you get up in the morning is not much fun. What is worse is that you start to let the BBT chart dictate your sex life. This is why though the BBT chart used to be a useful method in the past, its utility is limited today, as newer and more accurate methods are available.

Endometrial Biopsy

After ovulation, the endometrium is prepared for the implantation of the fertilized egg by the progesterone secreted by the corpus luteum. In order to determine whether or not ovulation is occurring normally, an endometrial biopsy may be done. During this procedure, a small amount of endometrium from inside the uterine cavity is extracted and sent for pathological examination under a microscope. This is a standard procedure usually done just before the period begins. It can be done in the doctor's clinic or in an operating theatre. No anesthesia or hospitalization is needed. However, discomfort is caused during the procedure (about as much as a severe menstrual cramp) and an analgesic can be taken a half-hour prior to the procedure to decrease this discomfort.

When examining the endometrial biopsy, the pathologist looks for the influence of the estrogen and progesterone hormones on the endometrial glands. If progesterone has been produced during that cycle, the endometrial glands show secretory changes. In fact, the effect of progesterone on the endometrium is so predictable, that the biopsy can be "dated", that is, the pathologist can predict on which day the next period will start! If there is a "lag" between the predicted day and the actual day, then such a lag suggests a luteal phase defect, which means that the production of progesterone is deficient. If no progesterone at all has been produced, then the endometrium will be reported as being proliferative (under the influence of only estrogen), which suggests that the cycle was anovulatory (i.e., ovulation did not occur in that cycle).

Curettage

A curetting used to be the commonest procedure done for infertile patients. In fact, a number of infertile patients still request that a curetting be done for them, since they feel that the procedure will clean out the "dirt" that they have accumulated in their uterus, and this will then allow them to conceive. This is an old wives' tale and is based on: "I know someone who got a baby after a curetting." The correct technical term for curetting is D & C (dilatation and curettage), which means that the cervix is stretched (dilated) and the uterine cavity scraped (curetted) to collect the endometrium. This is an obsolete procedure for an infertile woman, and can actually be harmful. The only use of a D&C is to provide endometrial tissue which can be examined under the microscope to see if the woman is ovulating or not. It has absolutely no fertility-enhancing role whatsoever. Since this endometrium can be obtained much more easily, safely and cheaply with an endometrial biopsy (in which only a strip of endometrium is removed), there should rarely be any need to do a D&C for an infertile woman. Patients have often had repeated D&Cs, and these can actually damage the cervix and even block the fallopian tubes, if infection occurs after surgery. The only possible role for a D&C today is when tuberculosis of the uterus is suspected.

Blood Tests for Progesterone

The progesterone level in the patient's blood may be measured to confirm that ovulation has taken place. Such a test is done on day 21 of the cycle (about one week after the presumed date of ovulation). A high progesterone level indicates that the corpus luteum is producing enough of the hormone and is good retrospective evidence that ovulation occurred. A very low level means that the cycle was most probably anovulatory. An intermediate level may suggest a luteal phase defect (in which the corpus luteum does not secrete enough progesterone).

Let us now discuss the symptoms and tests which can be used in order to determine when you ovulate.

Cervical Mucus (Billing's Method)

By checking your cervical mucus daily, as described in the chapter on the cervical factor, you can determine when you ovulate. Just before ovulation, your cervical mucus is thin, profuse, clear and stretchy, like raw egg white. After ovulation, the mucus becomes thick, tacky, scanty and sticky. You can learn to appreciate this change in your mucus (by seeing and feeling it) and this allows you to predict when ovulation occurs quite accurately.

Abdominal Pain

Approximately 25% of women may experience a pain on one side of the abdomen that is associated with ovulation. This pain is called *Mittelschmerz* (a German word, which means midcycle pain) and is usually related to the release of an egg from the rupturing follicle. It is a good idea to mark the date when it occurs since this information is helpful in determining when ovulation occurs.

The Role of Ultrasound

The egg develops within a follicle in the ovary. This follicle is a thin-walled structure which contains fluid and the egg is attached to its wall. Usually, only one follicle matures and develops every month. This follicular growth can be measured using a painless procedure called ultrasound, usually done with a vaginal probe, which projects an image of the ovary onto a screen. The follicle appears as a circular, fluid-filled bubble on the screen, and can be seen when it is about 7 mm to 8 mm in size. It grows at the rate of about 1 mm to 2 mm per day, and is ready for ovulation when it measures 18 mm to 25 mm in diameter. Following ovulation, the follicle usually disappears from the scan picture completely and this provides the best evidence of ovulation. Often, at the same time, fluid can also be detected in the abdomen behind the uterus – this is the follicular fluid which is released when the follicle ruptures. Defects detectable by ultrasound are follicles that do not grow at all, or do not grow to an appropriate size, or occasionally follicles that do not rupture at the appropriate time (*luteinized unruptured follicle syndrome*). Since ultrasound allows assessment of follicular development, it is especially useful for patients having timed intercourse or having ovulation regulated with fertility drugs. It is usually done on a daily basis, from about the 11th day of the cycle.

Follicle tracking on ultrasound usually takes about 5 minutes to perform. No prior preparation is needed except that the bladder must be emptied before the scan. Ask the doctor to show you the picture of the follicle on the monitor. You should be able to see the growth of the follicle and its rupture for yourself on the screen!

Older ultrasound machines used abdominal probes. These probes require that the patient have a full bladder, so that the sound waves can reach the ovary. Not only are they much more uncomfortable for the patient (who has to sit waiting till the bladder is almost bursting) but the quality of the pictures is also much poorer as compared to the vaginal scan.

Commercially Available Ovulation Prediction Kits

Ovulation prediction test kits are available abroad (and also in India at a few chemists) over the counter. These kits test for the hormone, LH (luteinizing hormone) which is produced in large quantities shortly before ovulation and can be detected in the urine. Once the LH surge has occurred, ovulation usually takes place within 12 to 44 hours. Urine testing is started about two days prior to the expected day of ovulation and continues until the test becomes positive. The urine should be collected at the same time every day and testing the first morning urine sample systematically is a good idea.

If your menstrual cycles are irregular, testing should be timed according to the earliest and latest possible dates of ovulation. For example, if your cycle ranges between 27 and 34 days, you could possibly ovulate between days 13 and 20. Therefore, testing should begin on day 11 and continue until ovulation is indicated or through day 20. The more frequent the testing, the better the chance of detecting ovulation accurately. Thus, there is an 80% chance of detecting ovulation after five days of testing and a 95% chance after ten days. Occasionally, ovulation may not occur in a particular cycle. If the ovulation prediction test has been timed and performed accurately and has not turned positive, you should discontinue testing and begin again during your next menstrual cycle. Persistent failure of the test to turn positive may indicate a problem with regard to ovulation.

OVULATION – NORMAL AND ABNORMAL

Once a test has registered positive, indicating that ovulation is about to take place, it is no longer necessary to continue testing. Remaining tests in a kit may be saved and used in the following menstrual cycle if pregnancy does not occur.

Ovulation prediction kits offer the advantage that they allow you to predict when ovulation will occur (and you can do them in the privacy of your own home!), thus maximizing the chances that intercourse can be timed at your most fertile period. However, such kits are expensive and some of them have very tedious and involved testing procedures, so that errors are not uncommon.

Blood Tests

The growing follicle secretes the hormone *estradiol* in increasing amounts and its blood level rises rapidly several days prior to ovulation. If ovulation is being induced through fertility drugs, estradiol blood tests may be done on a daily basis in order to determine if the developing follicles are growing properly. Normally, the estradiol blood levels should increase rapidly (as a rule of thumb, they double every 24 hours).

Since the luteinizing hormone (LH) blood level rises rapidly just before ovulation (this is called the LH surge), frequent blood samples for measuring the LH level can also be taken a few days prior to the anticipated time of ovulation in an attempt to predict when the follicle is mature and ready for ovulation.

Abnormal Ovulation

Abnormalities of ovulation may appear in several forms. Menstrual cycles shorter than 21 days or longer than 35 days are often associated with anovulation (absent ovulation). In addition, patients may skip menstrual periods for time intervals of three months or more and this condition is called oligomenorrhea (infrequent periods).

If the periods stop entirely, such a condition is called amenorrhea.

Many hormonal systems work together to produce regular menstrual periods, and the blood levels of the hormones that make up these systems need to be tested in order to determine the reason for the ovulatory disorder.

The hormone blood tests, which are usually done on the third day of your cycle, include the following:

The FSH level: The FSH level provides an idea of the number of eggs remaining in the ovaries – it is a crude index of the ovarian functional reserve. A high FSH level suggests that ovarian function has either failed or has started to fail. If the FSH level is very high (in the menopausal range) then the diagnosis is ovarian failure. If the level is on the border line, then some doctors will go in for a *clomiphene-stimulated FSH level test*, which allows for an earlier diagnosis of failing ovaries. On the other hand, a low FSH level suggests *hypogonadotropic hypogonadism*. This seemingly verbose term simply means that the ovary is not working properly because of inadequate production of FSH by the pituitary gland. However, in most anovulatory patients, the FSH level will be in the normal range, and this can be reassuring.

The LH level: LH is the other gonadotropin hormone produced by the pituitary gland and the LH level provides much the same information that the FSH level does. Another useful test is the LH : FSH ratio which is normally 1:1. If, however, the LH level is much higher than the FSH level, this finding suggests a diagnosis of polycystic ovarian disease.

Thyroxine and TSH: These test for the thyroid function. The thyroxine level is high in patients with overactive thyroid glands (hyperthyroidism). In patients with decreased thyroid function (hypothyroidism), the TSH level is increased.

Prolactin: Prolactin is a hormone produced by the pituitary gland. High prolactin levels (hyperprolactinemia) lead to the absence of ovulation.

Ovarian Failure

Ovarian failure is a disease in which the ovaries fail to produce eggs. This disease is uncommon, occurring in only about 10% of women whose periods do not occur at all, a condition called amenorrhea (absence of periods). Ovarian failure may be genetic (for example, in girls with Turner's syndrome, a chromosomal disorder) or may be acquired (for example: following radiation or chemotherapy for cancer; surgery to remove the ovaries for treating ovarian cancer or severe endometriosis; autoimmune ovarian failure; or for unexplained reasons). Ovarian failure is diagnosed by finding a high FSH level. In such patients, it is usually not possible to stimulate ovulation, because they do not have any eggs, and they suffer a premature menopause. The only effective medical treatment for most of these patients is the use of egg donation for IVF or GIFT. However, in a very small proportion of these patients, ovulation can resume spontaneously.

Induction of Ovulation

What forms of treatment are available for inducing ovulation?

The most commonly prescribed medicines for the induction of ovulation include the following: clomiphene citrate, human menopausal gonadotropin (HMG) and follicle-stimulating hormone (FSH), HCG (human chorionic gonadotropin), bromocriptine, GnRH (gonadotropin-releasing hormone) and GnRH analogue.

For women with hypogonadotropic hypogonadism (low FSH and LH levels), the treatment of first choice is HMG. This is an effective replacement therapy and excellent pregnancy rates can be achieved in these women.

For women affected by hyperprolactinemia, the drug of first choice is bromocriptine.

For most other women, the drug of first choice is clomiphene – the "workhorse" of ovulation induction. If this drug does not work, then HMG is resorted to.

Poor responders to HMG can be treated with GnRH analogues in conjunction with HMG; or by adding a hormone called the human growth hormone (HGH).

HCG (human chorionic gonadotropin) is given to trigger off the release of the egg.

In patients with high androgen levels (high blood levels of male hormones), dexamethasone can be used as an adjunct, since this suppresses androgen production.

Often, ovulation induction requires a considerable investment of time, money, energy and emotion before a satisfactory response is achieved. After all, each woman is different from the other and there can be no standard "formulae". Careful monitoring of the response to ovulation induction is the key to therapy and this usually involves daily ultrasound scans and/or blood tests. It is often a tedious process, which may involve "trial and error", to tailor the therapy to the individual patient's ovulatory response. However, with the present advances in medical science, correcting ovulatory dysfunction is one of the most rewarding and successful of infertility treatments.

13

Polycystic Ovarian Disease (PCOD)

PATIENTS SUFFERING FROM POLYCYSTIC ovarian disease (PCOD) have small multiple cysts in their ovaries. These cysts occur when the regular changes of a normal menstrual cycle are disrupted. The ovary is enlarged; and it produces excessive amounts of androgenic and estrogenic hormones. This excess, along with the absence of ovulation, may cause infertility. Other names for PCOD are polycystic ovarian syndrome (PCOS) or the Stein-Leventhal syndrome.

Diagnosis

PCOD can be easy to diagnose. The typical medical history is that of irregular menstrual cycles, which are unpredictable and can be very heavy, and the need to take hormonal tablets (progestins) to induce a period. Patients suffering from PCOD are often obese and may have hirsutism (excessive facial and body hair), as a result of the high androgen levels.

The diagnosis can be confirmed by vaginal ultrasound, which shows that both the ovaries are enlarged, with a bright central stroma and multiple small cysts. Typically, blood levels of hormones reveal elevated levels of androgens [a high dehydroepiandrosterone sulphate (DHEA-S) level], a high LH level, and a normal FSH level.

We don't really understand what causes PCOD. However, obesity can lead to PCOD because fatty tissues are hormonally active and they produce estrogen, which disrupts ovulation. Overactive adrenal glands can also produce excess androgens, and cause PCOD.

Treatment

Treatment of PCOD in infertile patients will usually focus on inducing ovulation to help them conceive.

Weight loss: For many patients with PCOD, weight loss is an effective treatment, but, of course, this is easier said than done! Look for a permanent weight loss plan. Referral to a dietician or a weight control clinic may be helpful. Crash diets are usually not effective.

Increasing physical activity is an important step in losing weight. Aerobic activities such as walking, jogging or swimming are advised. Try to find a partner to share your exercise schedule, so that you can help each other to keep going.

Ovulation induction: For ovulation induction, the drug of first choice is clomiphene which is often combined with low doses of dexamethasone, a steroid which suppresses androgen production from the adrenal glands. If clomiphene does not work, HMG can be used. Some doctors prefer to use pure FSH for inducing ovulation in PCOD patients because they have abnormally high levels of LH. Difficult patients may also need a combination of a GnRH analogue (to stop the abnormal release of FSH and LH from the pituitary) and HMG to induce ovulation successfully.

Surgery: In rare cases, it may not be possible to achieve ovulation with clomiphene or HMG. Some of these patients may be treated with ovarian surgery called *wedge resection* in order to help them to ovulate. The removal of the abnormal ovarian tissue in the wedge breaks the vicious cycle of PCOD, helping ovulation to occur. While wedge resection used to be a popular treatment option, the risk of inducing adhesions around the ovary as a result of this surgery has led to the operation being used only as a last resort.

A recent treatment option uses laparoscopy to treat some patients affected by PCOD. During operative laparoscopy, a laser or cautery is used to drill multiple holes through the thickened ovarian capsule. Destroying the abnormal ovarian tissue (much like a mini wedge resection) helps to induce ovulation.

With the currently available treatment options, successful treatment of infertility is usually possible in the majority of patients with PCOD.

14

The Cervical Factor

Normal Cervical Mucus

CERVICAL MUCUS IS A JELLY-LIKE substance produced by tiny glands in the cervix called *cervical crypts*. It has a protective function and may prevent bacteria from getting into the uterine cavity. The mucus changes predictably and cyclically during the menstrual cycle. During the first half of the cycle, before ovulation, when the estrogenic hormones are produced in ever-increasing amounts, the mucus produced by the cervical glands becomes watery, copious, clear and stretchy. Sperm can penetrate this watery mucus easily, and when intercourse takes place, sperm swim through this mucus rapidly into the uterus.

After ovulation, the quality of the mucus changes because the corpus luteum of the ovary now starts to make the hormone progesterone. Mucus produced under the influence of progesterone is thicker, stickier and its quantity is reduced. Sperm cannot swim through this mucus, and it forms a barrier to sperm entry into the uterine cavity.

Even if intercourse occurs at the time when the cervical mucus is at its most favourable, only about one in every 2000 sperm enters the mucus. The rest of the sperm remain in the vagina, where they die quickly, because of the acidic pH of the vaginal medium. Those sperm that have entered the mucus can survive there for long periods; certainly for several days after intercourse. Once in the cervical mucus, the sperm steadily swim upwards from it into the uterus over a period of 48 to 72 hours. Thus, the cervical mucus acts as a sperm reservoir, to be banked on if intercourse does not take place at ovulation. This is why you don't need to have sex every day in order to conceive! The cervical mucus also acts as a filter, and allows only the best sperm to swim through it into the uterus and up towards the egg present in the fallopian tube.

Observing the Mucus

Mucus flows from the cervix down the walls of the vagina and can be observed when it reaches the vulva. You can learn to observe the changes in your mucus by becoming aware of the wet, lubricative feeling produced by the mucus, and by observing the mucus itself at the vulva. This is called the Billing (fertility awareness) method, and is very useful in allowing you to determine when you ovulate.

You need to chart what the mucus looks like and feels like daily, from the day your bleeding stops. You will find the mucus present at your vaginal opening -- the vulva. Remember, you do not need to feel inside the vagina; this will simply confuse the picture, because the vagina is always moist. It is the vulva which is the mucus (fertility) monitor.

In a typical 28-day menstrual cycle, at the end of bleeding, the sensation you experience is one of dryness and no mucus is seen or felt. In some women, there is some mucus, but it is thick, sticky, and scanty. This is the basic infertile pattern of dryness and lasts for two to three days. Once this is over, you may notice a feeling of moistness at the vulva and the mucus will change in appearance and feel. It becomes thinner, clearer, more profuse and stretchy, like raw egg white. This fertile-type mucus produces a slippery wet lubricative sensation at the vulva. The last day of this fertile-type mucus (that is, the last day when the mucus looks stringy or feels wet, or the vulva feels lubricative) is called the peak of fertility, because it is the most fertile day of the cycle. You will know it is the last day only in retrospect; and after this, the mucus becomes thick, cloudy and sticky again. It is important to realize that the peak day is not necessarily the day of the highest mucus formation; it is simply the last day that the mucus discharged has fertile characteristics. Ovulation usually occurs with 24 hours of the peak mucus signal. Therefore, these are the best days to have intercourse in order to maximize the chances of conception.

Problems with the Cervical Mucus

In some women, the cervical mucus may prevent the sperm from moving freely into the uterus. Such a barrier may be because of the following reasons:

- There is not enough of the mucus to allow the sperm to swim easily.
- The mucus is too thick and sticky.
- The mucus is not compatible with the husband's sperm.

Tests on the Cervical Mucus

Problems related to cervical mucus usually exhibit no symptoms. Consequently, tests need to be done to assess whether the mucus is normal or not.

The doctor examines the cervix and the cervical mucus daily from about the tenth day of the period. The mouth of the cervix is graded, depending upon how open it is and the mucus is graded for its amount; its stretchability (*Spinnbarkeit*) and its ability to *fern*. For the ferning test, a small drop of mucus is placed on a glass slide and allowed

THE CERVICAL FACTOR

to dry. It should crystallize, and form pretty branch-like patterns under the microscope, which look like fern leaves. These scores are added to give an *Insler mucus score*. Healthy cervical mucus is profuse in volume; very stretchable (up to 10 cm in length); and ferns easily.

The *postcoital test* (PCT) is one of the oldest tests for investigating infertility and has been utilized for well over 100 years. Timing the PCT is critical, and it must be done in the preovulatory period, when the mucus is profuse and clear. The gynecologist examines a small sample of the cervical mucus under a microscope a few hours after sexual intercourse. The mucus is sucked painlessly from the cervical canal during an internal examination. Most doctors feel that the best time to carry out this test is about 6 to 24 hours after sex, but this timing is not critical. The test is said to be positive if many normal live sperm are seen swimming in the mucus sample. The sperm should be swimming in a fairly straight line and reasonably vigorously. A positive PCT is very reassuring and implies that:

1. The husband is likely to be producing enough normal sperm.
2. Intercourse results in semen being deposited in the vagina.
3. The cervical glands are healthy and produce good mucus.
4. Sufficient estrogen is being produced before ovulation, suggesting that ovulation is normal.
5. There are no antibodies in the mucus hostile to the sperm.

What if the PCT is negative (that is, no sperm are seen in the mucus or they are all dead)? Some of the reasons for a negative test are:

- The PCT has not been done at the best possible time. For example, the PCT may have been done

too early or too late in the cycle. Wrong timing is the commonest reason for a negative test and can even cause repeatedly negative tests.
- Ovulation did not occur during the month of the test — perhaps because of the strain or stress of making "love to order".
- The sperm count has been poor. Obviously, men with persistently low sperm counts, or those with poor motile sperm, may be responsible for a negative PCT.
- There may be an abnormality of the cervix; for example, chronic infection in the cervix may prevent production of adequate mucus; and some women with a scarred cervix may not produce enough mucus.
- The cervix may be producing antibodies to the sperm.
- Medications such as clomiphene, tamoxifen, progesterone and danazol — all drugs used for infertility problems — could have interfered with the production of good mucus.

Remember that a negative test is meaningful only if it is repeatedly negative even under perfect conditions.

If the mucus quality is good but the postcoital test is repeatedly bad, an *in vitro* mucus penetration test, or sperm invasion test, can be performed. This test is performed simply by putting a drop of freshly removed mucus next to a drop of freshly ejaculated semen on a microscope slide. The interface between the two drops is examined after some time, and it is then possible to see if the sperm are penetrating the mucus and swimming actively in it. If such activity does not occur, then it is likely that there is some form of immunity problem between the sperm and the mucus, and further tests should be conducted to examine this possibility.

THE CERVICAL FACTOR

Cross-over testing can be performed using the patients' mucus and semen in various combinations with donor mucus and donor semen. Such testing will show if the problem lies with the sperm or the mucus.

Another simple test for antisperm antibodies in the mucus is called the *sperm cervical mucus contact test* (SCMC for short), where the sperm and mucus are mixed together. If, under the microscope, the sperm are observed to be shaking in a characteristic way, this means that there are antibodies present.

Cervical problems can be corrected depending upon the specific cause. For example, if the reason for the poor mucus is lack of ovulation, then ovulation can be induced; if the reason is cervical infection, then this infection can be treated by cauterizing or freezing the abnormal cervical tissue, so that this tissue is shed, and is then replaced by healthy cervical glands. If the mucus is thick or viscous, then, occasionally, this condition can be treated by cough medicines (expectorants, which make the mucus thin). If the mucus is scanty, then donor mucus (from another woman) can be used or mucus production can be enhanced by supplemental low-dose estrogens.

For resistant cervical problems, the easiest solution may be to bypass the cervix entirely, by injecting the sperm directly into the uterus – a procedure called "intrauterine insemination".

Sometimes, the problem could be one of cervical immune hostility to the sperm; that is, there are antisperm antibodies in the mucus which are killing the sperm. For this condition the outlook is now more hopeful.

- Some doctors recommend that the woman avoid contact with sperm for a specific period of time. Such a step may cause the antibodies to disappear because their production is no longer being stimulated by repeated exposure to the antigen. The couple can have sex, but the husband must

wear a condom so that the sperm don't come in contact with the cervix. This course may be recommended for a period six months, until the antibodies have disappeared. This treatment is rarely suggested nowadays!
- Some doctors have tried inseminating the husband's washed sperm directly into the uterus, thus bypassing the cervix (and therefore the site of the antibodies). This treatment of intrauterine insemination has had limited success in some clinics but there is doubt about its value. This is because if antibodies are being produced, they may be present not only in the mucus, but also in the uterine cavity.
- Steroids may be given to prevent production of antibodies. To be effective they have to be given in high doses and this may cause serious side effects. However, such treatment is in the experimental stage and is not always effective.
- IVF can be tried. The presence of antisperm antibodies in the cervix will not interfere with *in vitro* fertilization and this could provide a treatment option for patients with intractable antibody problems.

15

Hirsutism—Excess Facial and Body Hair

HIRSUTISM REFERS TO THE GROWTH of long, coarse hair on the face and body of women in a pattern similar to that found in men. Besides being cosmetically distressing, hirsutism may also signal the presence of a hormone imbalance or a hormone-producing tumour.

Normal Hair Growth

Each hair grows from a follicle deep in the skin. As long as these follicles are not completely destroyed, hair will continue to grow even if the shaft, which is the part of the hair that appears above the skin, is plucked or removed.

Adults have two types of hair, namely, *vellus* and *terminal*. Vellus hair is soft, fine, colourless, and usually short. In most women, vellus hairs grow on the face, chest, and back and give the impression of "hairless" skin. Terminal hairs are the longer, coarser, darker, and sometimes curly variety that grow on the scalp, pubic, and armpit areas in both adult men and women. The facial and body hair in men is mostly of the terminal type.

What Causes Hirsutism?

Most often, excess facial and body hair is the result of abnormally high levels of androgens (the male hormones) in the blood. Androgens are present in both men and women, but men have much higher levels. These hormones cause hairs to change from vellus to terminal. Once a vellus hair has been transformed to the coarser terminal hair, it usually does not change back. Androgens also cause terminal hairs to grow faster and thicker. Both the ovaries and the adrenals produce androgens. To some degree, estrogen and progesterone (the female hormones) prevent the effect of androgens.

The following conditions can lead to high androgen levels, which, in turn, can cause hirsutism.

Genetics

Very obvious family and racial characteristics are noticeable in patients with hirsutism. In some women, the skin is very sensitive to even low levels of androgens and their follicles produce primarily terminal (coarse and dark) hairs. If your mother, grandmother or sister has experienced the disorder, then you are at a greater risk of developing it.

Polycystic Ovarian Syndrome

This syndrome is the commonest reason for hirsutism in infertile women. The polycystic ovarian syndrome causes the ovaries to develop many small cysts and to overproduce male hormones. The disorder is often associated with hirsutism, irregular ovulation, menstrual disturbances and obesity.

Ovarian Tumours

On rare occasions, androgen-producing ovarian tumours cause hirsutism. When this happens, hirsutism progresses rapidly and may even cause virilization, a condition in which the woman starts developing masculine characteristics, such as a deep voice and an enlarged clitoris. An ovarian mass may be detected during a pelvic examination.

Adrenal Disorders

The adrenal glands, which are located just above each kidney, also produce androgens. The most common disease of the adrenal gland that can result in hirsutism is an inherited disorder called *late onset adrenal hyperplasia*. Adrenal tumours and other adrenal diseases, such as Cushing's disease, can also cause overproduction of androgens.

Determining the Cause

When trying to ascertain the cause of hirsutism, several blood tests need to be done to measure androgen levels. These tests are done by radioimmunoassay in specialized laboratories, and include determining the levels of: testosterone; androstendione; 17-hydroxyprogesterone; and DHEA-S (dehydroepiandrosterone sulphate). These tongue-twisters are simply the chemical names of androgens produced in the body. Which particular hormone level is increased will tip off the doctor as to where the problem lies – whether in the ovaries or in the adrenal glands. A pelvic ultrasound, CT scan, or special X-ray studies may also need to be done to detect ovarian or adrenal tumours. Hormone suppression or stimulation tests which further evaluate the function of the ovaries and adrenal glands may also be required. During these tests, blood is measured for hormone levels both before and after the administration of a specific hormone medication. For example, the ACTH (adrenocorticotropic hormone) stimulation test is conducted in order to check for the presence of late onset adrenal hyperplasia.

Treatment

Of course, the priority will be to correct the problem of infertility. Thus, for example, if the problem of hirsutism is a result of anovulation because of the polycystic ovarian syndrome, the primary goal will be to induce ovulation.

Low doses of steroids called dexamethasone or prednisone may also be prescribed if the adrenal gland is overactive. The steroid is usually taken at bedtime and serves to suppress production of the ACTH hormone which stimulates the adrenal gland, thus decreasing the production of androgens by the adrenal gland.

Hormone treatment may prevent new hairs from developing. However, it usually takes many years for the excess hair to develop, and a significant decrease in the rate of hair growth will not be seen for at least six months after the commencement of hormone treatment. Once a hormone treatment has proven to be effective, it may be continued indefinitely. However, terminal hairs that are already present will not fall out or disappear with hormonal therapy and must be removed by other means.

Cosmetic Therapy

For temporary hair removal, many women with mild hirsutism pluck off the unwanted hairs. Waxing, another alternative, is essentially the same as plucking.

Depilating (hair-removing) agents are chemicals that dissolve the hair shafts on both facial and body hair and may also be used to remove unwanted hair. These chemicals can cause irritation, and facial skin is particularly sensitive.

Shaving is probably the simplest and safest temporary hair removal procedure. Although frequently required, it is virtually painless and seldom produces side effects. Contrary to popular belief, shaving does not make hair grow faster. An electric razor produces less skin irritation than a blade.

Electrolysis is the only permanent way to remove unwanted hair. During this procedure, a very fine needle is placed next to the hair shaft and inserted into the follicle. A mild electric current is sent through the needle which permanently kills the hair follicle. It is not possible to use this technique to remove hairs from very large areas of the body because each hair must be treated individually. In addition, this technique, although quite effective, is expensive, time consuming, and moderately uncomfortable. If hormonal therapy is being started, it is best to delay electrolysis for at least six months so that the growth of new terminal hairs will be reduced.

16

Endometriosis – The Silent Invader

ENDOMETRIOSIS IS A COMMON DISORDER that affects many women of reproductive age. It occurs when the normal endometrial tissue (i.e., the lining of the uterus) grows outside the uterus. This misplaced tissue may implant itself and grow anywhere within the abdominal cavity.

Many specialists feel that severe endometriosis is more likely to be found in infertile women who have delayed pregnancy, and, for this reason, the condition is sometimes labelled a "career woman's disease".

Endometrial tissue, whether it is inside or outside the uterus, responds to the estrogen and progesterone produced by the ovaries during the reproductive cycle. Under the influence of the hormones, the misplaced tissue grows and swells, and when hormonal levels drop, the tissue may bleed. Unlike the normally situated endometrium, which is shed from the body as the menstrual discharge, the misplaced tissue (and blood) have no outlet. They remain in the abdominal cavity and irritate the surrounding tissue.

Endometriosis is highly unpredictable. Some women may have just a few isolated implants that never spread or grow, while, in others, the disease may spread throughout the pelvis. Endometriosis irritates surrounding tissue and may produce web-like growths of scar tissue called adhesions. The scar tissue can bind the pelvic organs and even cover them entirely. Many women who have endometriosis experience few or no symptoms. However, in some women, endometriosis may cause severe menstrual cramps, pain during intercourse, and infertility.

Endometriosis is a disease which has been called an "enigma wrapped inside a mystery", and there is a lot about it that we do not understand as yet.

What Causes Endometriosis?

Several theories exist as to how endometriosis begins. One possibility is retrograde menstruation, i.e., the backward flow of the menstrual discharge through the fallopian tubes into the pelvis. According to this theory, the endometrial cells may be implanted on the ovaries or elsewhere in the pelvic cavity.

What Does Endometriosis Look Like?

Early implants look like small, flat dark patches or flecks of blue or black paint sprinkled on the pelvic surfaces. These patches may remain unchanged, become scar tissue or spontaneously disappear over a period of months. Endometriosis may invade the ovary, producing blood-filled cysts called "endometriomas". With the passage of time, the blood darkens to a deep, reddish brown or tarry colour, giving rise to the description "chocolate cyst". These cysts may be smaller than a pea or larger than a grapefruit.

In some cases, bands of fibrous tissue called adhesions may bind the uterus, tubes, ovaries, and nearby intestines together. The endometrial tissue may also grow into the walls of the intestine; although it may invade neighbouring tissue, endometriosis is not a cancer.

What Are the Symptoms?

Progressively increasing dysmenorrhea (period pains or menstrual cramping) may be a symptom of endometriosis.

This symptom is caused by contractions of the uterine muscle initiated by prostaglandins released from the endometrial tissue. A puzzling feature of endometriosis is that the degree of pain that it causes is not related to the extent of the disease. Some women with extensive disease feel no pain at all. A woman affected by endometriosis may notice that, as the disease progresses, her periods become more painful or that the pain begins earlier or lasts longer.

Endometriosis can cause pain during intercourse, a condition known as *dyspareunia*. The thrusting motion of the penis can produce pain in an ovary bound by scar tissue to the top of the vagina or in a tender nodule of endometriosis.

Most women who have endometriosis report no bleeding irregularities. Occasionally, however, the disease is accompanied by vaginal bleeding at irregular intervals or by premenstrual spotting.

How does endometriosis cause infertility? The relationship between mild (early) endometriosis and infertility is controversial. Sometimes, in some patients, the endometriosis may be coincidental and unrelated to the fertility problem. In these patients, other factors may be involved in the infertility, such as poor quality sperm or ovulation disorders, and the endometriosis is merely a "red herring". Some women who have the condition are able to conceive, while others may be infertile due to endometriosis or a combination of factors.

The disease may hinder conception in various ways, especially when it is severe. Endometriosis may inflame surrounding tissue and spur the growth of scar tissue or adhesions. Bands of scar tissue may bind the ovaries, fallopian tubes, and intestines together and thus interfere with the release of eggs from the ovaries or with the ability of the tube to pick up the egg. Rarely, severe endometriosis may cause the tubes to become blocked. The presence of chocolate cysts in the ovary may also impair ovulation.

Diagnosis

Endometriosis *cannot* be diagnosed from symptoms alone. While a physician may suspect the disease if an infertile woman complains of severe menstrual cramps or pain during intercourse, many patients afflicted with the condition report no discomfort at all. The diagnosis thus can be confirmed only by a laparoscopy.

Laparoscopy enables the doctor to look inside the pelvis and inspect carefully the reproductive organs so as to confirm the presence of endometriosis. In fact, since endometriosis is often without symptoms, many doctors advise laparoscopy as part of the diagnostic study for all infertile women.

Looking through the laparoscope, the surgeon can observe the surface of the uterus, tubes, ovaries, and other pelvic organs. He can visually confirm the presence of the endometriosis and gauge its extent. If desired, a small piece of tissue can be removed for microscopic examination (biopsy). Early endometriosis can easily be missed if the laparoscopy is not performed carefully. The entire ovary should be inspected meticulously; and if it is found to be enlarged, it should be punctured to look for chocolate cysts.

In some cases, the surgeon may decide to treat the endometriosis during laparoscopy itself. If so, he makes other small abdominal incisions through which additional instruments are introduced for operative laparoscopy. The surgeon may then vaporize the lesions with a laser beam or destroy them with an electric current using a diathermy machine.

Other imaging technologies, such as ultrasound, computerized tomography or magnetic resonance imaging may be used to get more information about the extent of the disease. However, these procedures are useful only for identifying endometriotic cysts in the ovary.

Hormone Medication

The goal of hormonal treatment is to simulate pregnancy or menopause, two natural conditions known to inhibit the disease. In each case, the normal endometrium is no longer stimulated to grow and regress with each monthly cycle, and menstruation ceases. The growth of misplaced endometrial tissue usually will be suppressed as well.

To simulate the hormonal environment of pregnancy, birth control pills are prescribed. To be effective against endometriosis, these pills must be taken continuously without pausing for withdrawal bleeding. This state is sometimes called "pseudopregnancy".

The hormone derivative danazol is the medication most frequently used to treat endometriosis. During treatment with danazol, high estrogen levels are reduced to low levels, which are characteristic of natural menopause. This state is sometimes called "pseudomenopause". Danazol is an expensive medication, which is usually prescribed for six months or more. Unfortunately, large endometriotic cysts of the ovary are generally resistant to the drug.

Analogues of GnRH, the gonadotropin-releasing hormone, are the newest class of hormones used for endometriosis treatment. These analogues switch off production of FSH and LH from the pituitary, thus inducing a menopausal state. These analogues can be given in the form of special injections called "depot preparations", which release small quantities of the drug daily, allowing administration at monthly intervals.

Pregnancy cannot occur during the course of medical therapy for endometriosis. However, it is hoped that treatment will cause the endometriosis to shrink sufficiently so that it will no longer interfere with conception after the treatment has been stopped.

Surgery

Treating endometriosis merely through medicines has definite limitations, especially for the infertile patient. Medication usually controls mild or moderate pain and may eliminate small patches of the disease. But large chocolate cysts in the ovary are less likely to respond to medicine, and drugs alone cannot remove scar tissue. This is why surgery may be needed to improve fertility by removing adhesions, lesions, nodules or endometriomas.

As described earlier, laparoscopy can be used as a therapeutic tool. For example, fluid can be drained; adhesions freed; small patches of endometriosis destroyed by using a laser beam or electrical current. Even large endometriomas can be removed through the laparoscope by a skilled surgeon. However, not all cases can be treated through the laparoscope. More extensive microsurgery may be required when the scar tissue is thick or involves delicate structures. Some patients need a combination of medical and surgical treatment.

Treatment cannot "cure" endometriosis, but can only control it. If an infertile woman afflicted with endometriosis fails to conceive even after medical and surgical treatment, *in vitro* fertilization may be an option.

Endometriosis is a disease affecting millions of women throughout the world. For many, the condition goes unnoticed. But for others, it demands professional attention, especially when fertility is impaired. The best strategy to maximize chances of conception is to select a specialist who is familiar with the latest developments in endometriosis management.

17

Ectopic Pregnancy

AN *ECTOPIC PREGNANCY* IS ONE WHICH develops outside the uterus. Most ectopics are found in the fallopian tube and these are called "tubal pregnancies". However, they can also occur at other pelvic sites which include the ovary, the abdomen, and the cervix.

Fertilization normally occurs in the outer half of the fallopian tube which is called the *ampulla*. The embryo is then propelled along the fallopian tube, by the coordinated beating of the cilia which line the tube, towards the uterus. An ectopic pregnancy occurs when the embryo gets stuck in the fallopian tube and is implanted here, instead of moving on to the uterus.

Ectopic pregnancy occurs once in every one hundred pregnancies.

The commonest cause of a tubal pregnancy is tubal damage, which most often occurs due to pelvic inflammatory diseases. If tubal damage is severe, the tube gets totally blocked, as a result of which the patient becomes infertile. However, in the case of less severe infection, the tube remains open, but the tubal lining gets damaged, as a result of which the cilia can no longer function effectively. Other reasons for tubal damage include tubal surgery, infection following IUCD insertion, and previous tubal pregnancy.

Infertile patients face an increased risk of having an ectopic pregnancy, but the reasons for this are still unclear. Perhaps the cause of their infertility is subtle tubal damage. There is also an increased risk of tubal pregnancy after IVF, since the embryo may sometimes migrate after embryo transfer from the uterine cavity to the fallopian tube. The risk of ectopics after GIFT is greater than after IVF.

Initially, an ectopic pregnancy may appear just as a normal pregnancy, with a missed menstrual period and symptoms such as sore breasts and nausea. However, there is often abnormal vaginal bleeding which may occur at the time of (or a little later than) the expected period. Often, this bleeding is mistaken for a period. Pain on the side of the ectopic occurs commonly and may be associated with a feeling of light-headedness. Making the diagnosis on clinical examination is difficult, and the only suspicious finding may be pain on internal examination. If the tube ruptures, the patient experiences severe abdominal pain, fainting and shock.

A tubal pregnancy used to be considered a catastrophe. Diagnosis was usually made only after the tube had ruptured, and emergency surgery was required to stop the bleeding and save the patient's life. Often, this meant removing the whole tube, which was often completely damaged. Consequently, the chances of a patient's conceiving after such surgery was markedly reduced.

Today, an ectopic pregnancy can be diagnosed very early using blood tests for HCG and through vaginal ultrasound. Both these tests need to be done simultaneously in order to interpret the results correctly. The beta-HCG test is a very specific "marker" for pregnancy. This blood test is very sensitive and, if negative, virtually excludes any risk of a significant ectopic pregnancy. A positive HCG level confirms that the patient is pregnant, but does not provide information about the site of the pregnancy. A vaginal ultrasound allows the doctor to locate the gestational sac of the early pregnancy. Occasionally, the sac may be seen outside the uterus, making a positive diagnosis of the ectopic pregnancy on sonography. Often, however, the sac cannot be seen clearly in ectopic pregnancies, especially if it is in an early stage. Then, both the scan and HCG levels need to be studied.

Another blood test which can be helpful is the determination of the serum progestoerone level, which is low in patients with ectopic pregnancies, as compared to normal pregnancies.

Sometimes, differentiating between an ectopic pregnancy and an early miscarriage can be difficult. In these cases, if a curettage shows that there is no pregnancy tissue in the uterus (as tested by histopathologic examination), then an ectopic pregnancy is suspected. The diagnosis can be confirmed by laparoscopy, if needed, which shows that the pregnancy is in the tubes, where it appears as a dark bluish bulge.

The major benefit of early diagnosis is that early treatment can be started, making it possible to save the tube and thus preserving fertility and increasing the chances of a normal pregnancy in the future. If the ectopic pregnancy is very early and the HCG levels low, one can choose to simply wait and watch and monitor the patient carefully with serial HCG levels. Often, the HCG levels will fall, meaning that the pregnancy is being reabsorbed by the body on its own and no treatment is needed. Medical treatment is also possible. Such treatment involves the use of the anti-cancer drug, methotrexate, which acts on the rapidly dividing cells of the tubal pregnancy and kills them, thus preventing the pregnancy from growing further.

Ultrasound-guided treatment can also be useful for treating tubal pregnancies which have not ruptured. This treatment involves the injection of toxic chemicals into the tubal pregnancy under ultrasound guidance. These chemicals kill the pregnancy, allowing the body to reabsorb it.

ECTOPIC PREGNANCY

Surgical treatment for early tubal pregnancies can be done through the laparoscope as well; with salpingotomy, the pregnancy can be selectively removed and the tube saved.

If the tube has ruptured, and blood has collected in the abdomen, then emergency surgery is needed. In such cases, the tube is often so badly damaged, that it has to be removed entirely. When this occurs, a couple not only mourns the loss of a pregnancy, but also the possible loss or reduction in their fertility. This sense of loss is accompanied by the discomfort and anxiety of the wife having to undergo an emergency operation.

What about the chances of getting pregnant after an ectopic pregnancy? Because tubal disease usually damages both the fallopian tubes, the chances of being infertile are increased. Also, the risks of having a repeat ectopic pregnancy are increased even if the other tube seems normal. However, about 60% of women who have had a tubal pregnancy the first time will have a normal pregnancy the next time without further treatment. Early testing during pregnancy to rule out a repeat ectopic pregnancy is absolutely essential!

If pregnancy does not occur within about a year of trying, then treatment is needed. Treatment options for fertility will depend upon the kind of surgery done for the ectopic pregnancy and upon the condition of the other tube. Often, a second-look laparoscopy is required in order to assess tubal status. Options may include the following: ovulation induction; tubal surgery; laparoscopic surgery; and even IVF.

Having faced an unsuccessful outcome the first time makes getting pregnant very stressful, especially if the tubal pregnancy ended in a rupture. However, with the right treatment, the chances of having a baby are quite good – after all, the fact that a pregnancy occurred (even though it was an ectopic) means that the eggs and sperm are in good working order!

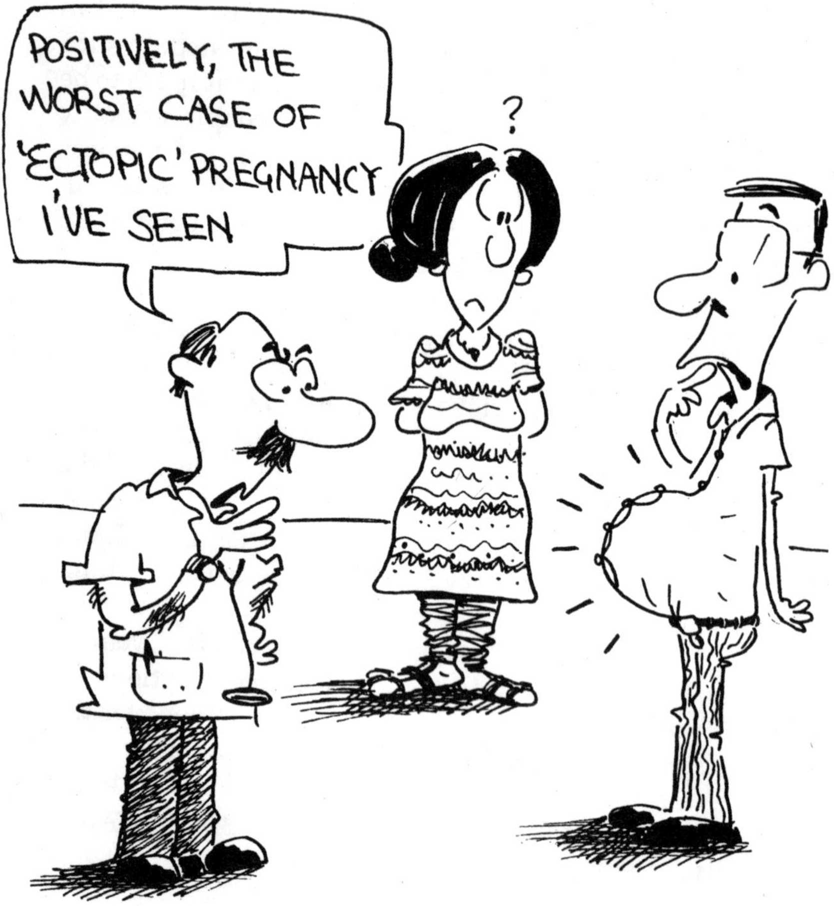
POSITIVELY, THE WORST CASE OF 'ECTOPIC' PREGNANCY I'VE SEEN
?

18

Unexplained Infertility

UNEXPLAINED INFERTILITY SIMPLY MEANS the doctors do not know why the couple is infertile — it is a confession of medical ignorance. Patients with unexplained infertility problems fall into two groups. The first group consists of those who really have no infertility problem whatsoever, but are just plain "unlucky". The other group has members who do have a reason for their infertility, but the reason is so elusive, that even with present-day medical technology, we cannot find it.

Infertility may be said to be "unexplained" in cases where the woman is ovulating regularly, has open fallopian tubes with no adhesions or endometriosis; the man has normal sperm production; and the postcoital test is positive. Intercourse must take place frequently, particularly around the time of ovulation, and the couple must have been trying to conceive for at least one year.

On the basis of aforementioned criteria, about 10% of all infertile couples have unexplained infertility. However, the percentage of couples classified as having unexplained infertility will depend upon the thoroughness of testing and the sophistication of medical technology.

The diagnosis in the case of unexplained infertility is one of exclusion, that is, one which is made only after all the tests have been performed and their results found to be normal. This is why, the frequency of this diagnosis will depend upon how many tests have been done by the clinic – the fewer the tests, the more frequent this diagnosis.

Possible causes of unexplained infertility are as follows:

1. *Tubal abnormalities*: It is possible that there may be a subtle defect in the mechanism by which the fimbria "pick up" the egg during ovulation; or else the cilia in the tube may not be functioning properly.

2. *Abnormal eggs*: A very small number of cases of unexplained infertility could be due to the persistent production of abnormal eggs. These eggs may have a deformed structure or chromosomal abnormalities.

3. *Trapped eggs*: In some cases, it appears that eggs are produced and matured correctly within the follicle, which then goes on to become a corpus luteum without, however, first bursting to release the egg. The egg is therefore effectively "trapped" inside the unbroken corpus luteum – and this is called a *luteinized unruptured follicle* (LUF) syndrome.

4. *Luteal phase abnormalities*: The luteal phase is that part of the cycle which follows after the egg has been released from the ovary. This phase may be inadequate in some way, and this is called a luteal phase defect.

The corpus luteum produces the hormone called progesterone, which is essential for preparing the endometrium to receive the fertilized egg. Several things can go wrong with progesterone production: the rise in output can be too slow; the level can be too low; or the length of time over which it is produced can be too short. Another possibility is a defective endometrium that does not respond properly to the progesterone.

Luteal phase defects can be investigated either by a properly timed endometrial biopsy or by monitoring the progesterone output by taking a number of blood samples on different days after ovulation and measuring the progesterone level in them.

5. *Immunological factors*: The immune system can react against the man's own sperm, and, as a result, kill them, immobilize them, or make them stick together. Women can also develop an immune reaction to the sperm, with the same result, thus preventing the sperm from reaching the egg. It is also possible that women can develop antibodies against the coating of their own eggs (the zona pellucida), and these can prevent sperm from binding to the zona.

6. *Infections*: Infection by certain disease particles has been shown to be responsible for some cases of unexplained infertility. A disease particle called "T-strain mycoplasma" may be present in a quantity that is not enough to show up in a clinical examination, but which, nevertheless, can cause infertility.

7. *Inability of sperm to penetrate eggs*: There is evidence to show that some men's sperm, although apparently adequate in every other way, are unable to get into the egg to fertilize it. The only way to make this diagnosis is by IVF; if donor sperm can fertilize the wife's eggs but the husband's sperm fail to do so, then the diagnosis is confirmed.

8. *Psychological factors*: Studies on infertile groups of men and women have produced contradictory findings about the importance of psychological factors in causing infertility. Emotional disturbances, undoubtedly, appear to be of some significance. Such a possibility is perfectly reasonable – after all, the whole hormonal cycle, with its delicate adjustments, is controlled from the brain. This is an area which needs further investigation, but it really is a "chicken and egg" kind of problem. Remember, that it is much commoner for the infertility to cause emotional stress, rather than for the emotional disturbance to result in infertility!

Has Anything Been Missed?

All previous tests undergone by the couple should be carefully reviewed by the doctor to ensure that the diagnosis is, in fact, "unexplained", and that no test has been omitted or missed. It may sometimes be necessary to repeat certain investigations. Thus, for example, if a previous laparoscopy has been done by a single puncture and been reported as normal, it may be necessary to repeat the laparoscopy with a double puncture, in order to look for early endometriosis.

How Can Unexplained Infertility Be Treated?

Remember, you still have a fairly good chance of getting pregnant on your own without any treatment at all! If no abnormality is found, your chance of getting pregnant without treatment within 3 years is about 1 in 3. Taking treatment helps to increase the chances of your conceiving—not only is the possibility of getting pregnant increased, but you are also likely to get pregnant more quickly.

The treatment of luteal phase defects is as controversial as their diagnosis. They can be treated by using clomiphene, which may help by augmenting the secretion of FSH and thus improving the quality of the follicle (and therefore the corpus luteum which develops from it). Direct treatment with progesterone can also help treat luteal phase abnormalities. The progesterone can be given either as injections or vaginal suppositories.

Today, with the availability of assisted reproductive technology, the chances of successful treatment are very high. Intrauterine insemination with superovulation is the simplest approach, since it increases the chances of the egg and sperm meeting; but some patients may also need GIFT and IVF. Further, IVF can be helpful, because it provides information about the sperm's fertilizing ability; GIFT, on the other hand, assures a higher pregnancy rate, and is applicable in these patients since they have normal fallopian tubes.

19

Secondary Infertility – Caught between Fertile and Infertile Worlds

FOR MOST PEOPLE, INFERTILITY CONJURES up the image of a couple without a child. But what about a couple who have borne a child, and now want to extend their family but find they are unable to do so?

Secondary infertility is the inability to conceive after one or more successful pregnancies. The medical causes are similar to those of primary infertility, and include sperm problems, tubal factors, endometriosis and ovulation difficulties. However, there are differences. For one thing, the couple would be older, and it may take the wife longer to conceive, which is why time is at a premium for them!

Moreover, emotional aspects that are unique have to be taken into consideration. The couple experiencing secondary infertility often finds it difficult to gain understanding or sympathy from family, friends and relatives. Since they have one child, most people assume that the couple will have no problem having another. Even other infertile couples offer little sympathy! Patients with primary infertility often resent couples who have a baby, and believe their own pain would disappear if only they too could bear one child. A common remark is : "You have one child, you should be grateful for that." Couples who are victims of secondary infertility, thus, are caught between two worlds, fertile and infertile – and are excluded from both!

Guilt and frustration are common emotional responses. The frustration is born out of surprise because the couple didn't think it would be difficult to conceive a second time (unless they had difficulty in achieving pregnancy the first time as well). However, just because they have achieved pregnancy once doesn't make them immune to all the illnesses which can cause infertility – tubes can get blocked and sperm counts can drop as time goes by!

Couples with secondary infertility who have undergone an elective abortion to terminate the first pregnancy and who cannot conceive a second time around have a very hard time coping with their feelings of guilt. They often feel they are being punished for their sin of rejecting the child when they could have had one.

Couples with a single child at home may also feel guilty. This guilt arises because they catch themselves feeling that one child isn't good enough for them and also for their inability to provide their child with a sibling.

The child of a secondarily infertile couple may also bring unwitting pressure on the parents by asking when he will have a baby brother or sister. This is especially difficult when the child is being asked by his friends why he doesn't have a baby brother or sister and then begs his parents for a baby.

Parents may become very overprotective, fearing that something may happen to the one child that they do have. They may also pin all their hopes on their one child, and may push him relentlessly to be a high achiever.

Many couples with secondary infertility choose never to take medical treatment. Often, this is because they are unsure about whether they do have a problem, and they keep on trying, hoping to "hit the jackpot" once again (after all, if they could do it once, why can't they do it again?).

What are the chances of a couple with secondary infertility conceiving with medical treatment? While the answer would depend upon their specific problem, their chances are really about the same as a couple with primary infertility. While the former couple have the benefit of having "proven" their fertility once, they usually have the handicap of increased age against them.

If the couple chooses to seek medical intervention, they also must decide what to tell their child about medical procedures. The presence of a child at home can make coping with the demands of infertility treatment much more difficult!

The financial burden of going in for treatment can also add to the couple's emotional stress and they may wonder if they shouldn't be spending the money on the child they already have rather than pursuing the hope of expanding their family.

Adoption can be a choice for some of these couples, but such an alternative is often more complicated because they worry about the possibility of "favouritism" and may also feel that it is unfair to their biological child to bring an adopted child into the family.

Coming to terms with secondary infertility is no easier than coming to terms with primary infertility and it's important that the family of the couple with secondary infertility share their feelings together and maintain a positive attitude.

20

Empty Arms – The Lonely Trauma of Miscarriage

AN EXTENDED DEFINITION OF INFERTILITY includes women who can conceive but cannot carry a pregnancy to the full term, that is, women who suffer repeated miscarriages or pregnancy failures.

The medical term for a miscarriage is an *abortion*. Most miscarriages start with vaginal bleeding which is initially slight and painless. This is called a " threatened abortion", because the pregnancy is threatened by the bleeding. This bleeding takes place from the mother, and is not fetal blood. About half the time, this bleeding stops spontaneously and causes no harm to the pregnancy. At this stage, the most useful test is an ultrasound scan (usually done with a vaginal probe). If a fetal heartbeat can be seen, this means that there is a 95% chance that the pregnancy will proceed normally. On the other hand, if the ultrasound scan shows that the fetus has not developed properly (and this includes patients with a blighted ovum or anembryonic pregnancy, when no fetus can be seen; or a missed abortion or intrauterine fetal death, when the fetus is seen but the heart is not beating) then nothing can be done to save the pregnancy. In these cases, the bleeding progresses, and the uterus starts contracting. The patient feels these contractions as painful cramps, and the mouth of the uterus (the cervix) opens. Such a situation is called an "inevitable abortion" (because it cannot be stopped). If a portion of the pregnancy tissue has already been expelled by the contractions, then this condition is called an "incomplete abortion".

In patients affected by blighted ovum, missed abortion, inevitable or incomplete abortion, the treatment is a uterine curettage (D & C) – a short surgical procedure which is performed to empty the uterus and remove the pregnancy tissue.

The medical definition of an abortion is the loss of a pregnancy before the fetus is viable, that is, before 20 weeks of pregnancy. Abortions which occur in the first 12 weeks of pregnancy are called "first trimester abortions" and those which occur between the 13th to 20th weeks are called "second trimester abortions".

The Magnitude of the Problem

Perhaps 20-30% of all women spot, bleed or suffer cramps during the first 12 weeks of their pregnancy, and about 10% miscarry. This figure may be an underestimate, because there are a number of women who miscarry unknowingly, thinking that their period has been late or heavy. It is very common for women to have one miscarriage during the first 12 weeks of their pregnancy. This mostly happens by chance and is not a sign that they have a health problem because most of them will probably have a healthy baby the next time that they get pregnant without any treatment.

If, however, a patient has suffered two or more miscarriages consecutively, this is called "repeated or habitual abortion". Now, although the risk of miscarrying again does go up, this risk is still quite small, and increases from the 15% risk a normal woman has to about 35%, which still means there is a 65% chance that she will *not* have a miscarriage again.

Facts and Fiction

Most women who miscarry do so only once. Their risk of miscarrying again is not increased and is the same as that of a normal woman's – about 15%.

Women who are over 35 years of age are more liable to miscarry.

There is an old saying that you cannot shake a good apple off a tree. Similarly, travelling, lifting weights and having sex do not threaten a healthy pregnancy.

If you've had a previous miscarriage, it is very normal to be frightened and worried during your next pregnancy. It is important to understand that exercise, working and intercourse do not increase the risk of pregnancy loss. Likewise, staying at home and resting in bed probably do not prevent miscarriage.

Causes

Repeated miscarriages can happen because of any of the following:

- Chromosomal abnormalities.
- Hormone imbalance.
- Physical illness.
- Polycystic ovarian syndrome.
- Immunity problems.
- Antiphospholipid antibodies.
- Problems in the uterus.
- Lifestyle of the woman.

Let's discuss these factors in detail.

Chromosomal Abnormalities

At least 60% of spontaneous miscarriages occur because of a chromosomal abnormality at the time of conception. This means that a genetically (chromosomally) defective sperm or ovum gives rise to a genetically abnormal fetus.

The miscarriage is Nature's defense mechanism, which aborts a defective fetus, rather than giving birth to a defective baby. Since most of these genetic defects are chance occurrences, the risk of the defects being repeated again in the next pregnancy is very small.

In order to establish the diagnosis of a genetic cause for repeated pregnancy loss, a *karyotype* (study of the chromosomes) of the fetal tissue (if available) may be done. A karyotype is expensive, and often the fetal cells fail to grow in culture, so that the study may not be possible. Moreover, since little can be done even if a defect is detected, it has little impact on patient management. However, it does provide an explanation for some patients who are affected by recurrent pregnancy loss.

In about 5% of couples, a chromosome abnormality found in one of the partners explains recurrent miscarriages. This abnormality is detected by doing a chromosomal study on the parents' blood. The commonest problem is a structural defect (break or loss of a piece of the chromosome; or a rearrangement of a bit of a chromosome).

If the karyotype is normal, then the patients can be reassured that the miscarriages were a chance genetic event, and they can feel comfortable continuing with their efforts to have a baby. However, if the karyotypes are abnormal, this is a permanent situation, which indicates an increased risk of miscarriage. Genetic counselling should be sought to discuss the degree of risk. Depending upon the individual problem, this risk may be anywhere from 25% to 100%. Since chromosomal rearrangement at conception (when the sperm fertilizes the egg) is a random event, there is little which can be done to treat this disorder. Options may include: continuing to try to conceive a baby naturally; adoption; donor eggs (if the wife is suffering from the genetic problem); or donor sperm (if the husband is affected by the genetic problem).

Hormone Imbalance

Patients may miscarry because they have a *luteal phase defect*, that is, the amount of progesterone hormone produced after the egg has been released is reduced. Progesterone is the hormone which supports the pregnancy. Progesterone helps implantation of the embryo in the uterus and if its production is deficient, there can be a problem with the embryo lodging itself in the uterine lining.

A luteal phase defect is suspected if the menstrual cycles are short, especially if the luteal phase (the time of the menstrual cycle between ovulation and the next menstruation) is shorter than 12 days.

The foregoing diagnosis can be confirmed by a blood test (a blood progesterone level, done one week after ovulation, is low) and an endometrial biopsy (which will show that the endometrium is "out of phase").

The doctor can help provide luteal support by prescribing progesterone during the last two weeks of the menstrual cycle after ovulation. If the woman is already pregnant, treatment may be done through vaginal suppositories of natural progesterone for the first 12 weeks of the pregnancy; or through progesterone injections intramuscularly. However, this treatment is controversial.

Illnesses

Health problems that can cause repeated miscarriages are:

- Endometriosis.
- Uncontrolled thyroid disease.
- Uncontrolled diabetes.
- Severe heart, liver or kidney disease.
- Systemic lupus erythematosus, an illness in which the woman produces antibodies against her own body tissues.

What about TORCH infections? Certain infections called TORCH (which stands for TOxoplasmosis, Rubella, Cytomegalovirus and Herpes), may be a cause for a single miscarriage, but are *not* a cause for repeated miscarriages. While a number of specialists will carry out these tests, and even start treatment based on the results, these tests are not worthwhile for patients who undergo habitual abortion.

Although infections of the uterine cavity (for example, due to mycoplasma) are frequently thought to be a cause of recurrent pregnancy loss, substantial proof of this aspect is lacking. Studies have, in fact, failed to indicate a greater incidence of infection in women with a history of miscarriage when compared to normal fertile women.

Polycystic Ovarian Syndrome

Exciting research done recently by Dr Howard Jacobs at the Middlesex Hospital, London, shows that the polycystic ovarian syndrome can also be a cause of recurrent miscarriages. In PCOS, the ovaries produce a large amount of the LH hormone. This hormone has a detrimental effect on the egg, so that, at the time of ovulation, the egg released is overripe and unhealthy. If such an egg is fertilized, the embryo is also likely to be unhealthy, and is consequently rejected by the body after 6-8 weeks as a miscarriage. The interesting point of these studies is that they tell us that we should also be focussing on what is happening at the time of fertilization – and not just on what goes on after the pregnancy has been implanted in the uterus. Problems pertaining to the eggs and sperm at the time of fertilization may only manifest themselves as a miscarriage of the fetus later on, but these problems are often overlooked by the doctor.

Immunity Problems

The immune system plays an important protective role in maintaining health throughout one's life by defending against infection. It "rejects" the foreign invaders (e.g., bacteria, viruses) which are recognized by the body as being "outsiders". It is now becoming evident that inappropriate activation of the mother's immune system may cause early first trimester miscarriages.

Current theory suggests that during a normal pregnancy, the fetus, which carries the father's foreign genes (and is therefore immunologically foreign to the mother) can, nevertheless, survive in the mother's uterus because of a special protection from the mother's immune system – the uterus is a "privileged" site. This is why the fetus is not "rejected" like other foreign tissues (such as kidney transplants) are. This means that in the normal course of events, the fertilized egg somehow stimulates a protective maternal immune response which allows implantation and growth. For certain couples, this protective response does not occur, and the maternal immune system rejects the father's foreign material in the fetus, resulting in miscarriage. At present, tests are available to check for such immunological rejection, but these tests are still in the experimental stage. Treatment also is still in the research phase, and includes sensitizing the mother to the father's genes, by injecting his blood cells into her skin, the theory being that exposure to the foreign cells would stimulate her immune system to provide the normal protective immune response when she gets pregnant.

Antiphospholipid Antibodies

Some women produce antibodies against the circulating substances that cause blood clotting. These antibodies are called *lupus anticoagulant* or *anticardiolipin* or *antiphospholipid antibodies*. They severely inhibit fetal development (by blocking off the blood supply to the fetus by causing clots in the maternal-fetal circulation) and cause miscarriages. Their presence can be detected by a blood test. Treatment is possible, either with low doses of aspirin (which decreases the clot formation) or with a steroid (prednisone, which suppresses the mother's abnormal immune system).

Problems in the Uterus

Miscarriages because of uterine problems usually occur after the twelfth week. These could be because of:

- A congenital abnormality of the uterus, which the woman is born with, but which does not cause any problems, until a pregnancy is attempted. Such a uterus (septate uterus, bicornuate uterus) cannot grow normally to hold and retain the pregnancy and the fetus is consequently expelled.
- Fibroids, which are growths of smooth muscle tissue inside the uterus. While most fibroids will not mar a pregnancy, if the fibroid is very close to the lining of the uterus (submucous fibroid), it will interfere with the implantation of the embryo in the uterus, and will cause its expulsion.
- Intrauterine adhesions (Ashermann's syndrome): These adhesions are uncommon, and are fibrous bands of scar tissue in the uterus, which interfere with implantation of the embryo. They may be formed after a uterine curettage (after an abortion) and can be diagnosed by hysteroscopy or hysterosalpingography. They can be removed by hysteroscopic surgery, allowing uneventful pregnancies in the future.
- Incompetent os, in which the cervix (mouth of the womb) is weakened: When the growing fetus presses on it, the weakened cervix opens, leading to expulsion of such a fetus. This condition may be congenital; or may result because of a cervical tear or injury during previous pregnancy or miscarriage; or could be a result of overenthusiastic surgical

dilatation of the cervix during previous surgery. The insertion of a cervical stitch (called the "Shirodkar stitch" after Dr Shirodkar of Bombay, who discovered this condition and invented the surgical operation to correct it), can be very effective. The cervical stitch is a simple surgical operation, usually done after 12 weeks of pregnancy after an ultrasound shows that the baby is healthy. This stitch helps by strengthening the weakened cervix. The stitch is removed two weeks before the baby is due, or when labour starts, whichever is first.

Diagnosis of the aforementioned anatomic defects can be made by hysteroscopy or hysterosalpingography. An ultrasound examination can suggest a problem exists, but usually cannot provide a definitive diagnosis.

Lifestyle of the Woman

If the woman is regularly exposed to toxic fumes and chemicals (for example, workers in chemical factories or nurses and anesthetists in operating rooms), these could damage the developing fetus (which is very sensitive to poisons) and cause a miscarriage. Recent studies show that even men exposed to environmental toxins can cause their partner to miscarry a fetus (presumably because their sperm are damaged by the toxins). Smokers, alcoholics and drug abusers also have an increased incidence of miscarriages.

The Emotional Aspects

Human society still tends to dismiss miscarriage complacently; it is a subject which is rarely discussed. A fetus for most people is a non-person and a miscarriage is a non-event. But, to the would-be parents, the developing fetus is a baby with an identity, specially if they have seen it on the ultrasound screen and heard its heart throbbing with a Doppler. When the child is lost, it is a bereavement and the sense of loss, tinged with pain, anger, isolation and depression, can be profound, especially when such a loss occurs after a long period of infertility.

After a miscarriage, it is normal to experience a period of grief. Find support from each other and from others who have had a similar experience. Healing does take place in time. Focus on getting through the grieving rather than on the suffering.

Your Next Pregnancy

After a miscarriage, making the decision to go in for another pregnancy is difficult. Collect as much information as possible to try to find out the possible causes of the loss and whether they might influence a future pregnancy.

If you have had two or more miscarriages, then tests are usually done to try to find a cause. These tests include the following:

- Hysterosalpingogram or hysteroscopy to make sure there are no defects in your uterus (womb).
- Blood tests, such as serum progesterone, to rule out a luteal phase defect.
- Blood tests for antiphospholipid antibodies (lupus anticoagulant).
- The VDRL (Venereal Diseases Research Laboratory) blood test, for sexually transmitted diseases.
- Karyotype, for you and your husband, to rule out chromosomal abnormalities.

Often many doctors will perform what is called a "TORCH" test, but this test is a waste of money for most patients, since it provides little useful information.

When to start the testing depends upon you. While few doctors would investigate a woman after a first miscarriage (since her chance of having a healthy pregnancy even without tests and treatment is higher than 85%), most would start a workup after two miscarriages.

Often, nothing is found, and such a situation can be very frustrating to both the doctor and the patient. But do remember that medical technology has its limitations, and we still do not know a lot about the early embryo and its development.

What about treatment? Sometimes it is possible to treat the underlying problem; for example, by inserting a cervical stitch to treat an incompetent os; or removing a uterine septum by hysteroscopic surgery. However, most treatment is "empirical" and is like shooting in the dark. Possible solutions could include: bed rest; progesterone injections and tablets; and uterine relaxants, such as Duvadilan, during pregnancy, though their real value is doubtful.

Often the only option is to try again. Remember, even if you have had three or more miscarriages, your chance of carrying the next baby to term is still more than 50% – even with no specific treatment, but just tender loving care!

Deciding when to start the next pregnancy is a question only you and your husband can answer. It takes a lot of courage and both of you need to be ready.

Your next pregnancy probably won't be as joyful as you would like it to be. Insist that your pregnancy be monitored carefully. Whenever the slightest problem occurs, you'll feel vulnerable and terrified, but don't panic.

Everyone will make suggestions about what you should do to make your pregnancy successful. This can be annoying, but remember people are doing it because they care! The easiest way to handle this is to listen to all views, but do what you and your doctor feel is best for you.

Your child birth experience can be bitter-sweet – memories surface about your loss, especially if you are at the same hospital. You probably will need to do some grieving in addition to celebrating the new life.

The experience of miscarriage will also affect your parenting. Bonding with your child may also be delayed because you feel the need to protect yourself from more sorrow; so you wait till you are certain that all is safe and sure with your baby. Moments of panic will occur when the baby is ill or too quiet or with someone else. You are also likely to treat your children as "extra special", and, consequently be less objective than other parents.

If you've experienced recurrent miscarriages, you may feel hopeless and confused regarding a positive pregnancy outcome. Remember that miscarriage is *not* an uncommon event. Your testing will focus on trying to find out the known causes of recurrent miscarriages. But knowledge of this problem is still limited, and no obvious cause has been detected in up to 50% of couples with repeated pregnancy loss. This can be very frustrating – to both the patient and the doctor. However, let us end this chapter on an optimistic note. The encouraging news is that the spontaneous cure rate is very high and successful treatment is available for treating certain uterine and endocrine causes. So even if your evaluation does not reveal a treatable cause and you do not undergo treatment, your chance of achieving a healthy pregnancy despite having had several miscarriages is still higher than 50%!

21

Understanding Your Medicines

YOU MUST BE KNOWLEDGEABLE ABOUT what medicines you are taking in order to combat your infertility, and why. It's easy for doctors to prescribe medicines, but it is your responsibility to be well-informed about them, so that you know exactly what to expect.

Medicines commonly used in infertility treatment include:

(a) Bromocriptine (Proctinal, B-crip, Parlodel).
(b) Clomiphene (Clomid, Fertyl, Ovofar, Serophene).
(c) Danazol (Ladogal, Danazol).
(d) HMG (Humegon, Pergonal, Nugon).
(e) FSH (Metrodin, Puregon).
(f) HCG (Pregnyl, Profassi, Life).
(g) GnRH analogues (Buserelin, Lucrin).

Bromocriptine

Bromocriptine is a drug which is used specifically to treat women with hyperprolactinemia, a condition in which women fail to ovulate because the pituitary is producing too much of the hormone called prolactin. Hyperprolactinemia is the cause of menstrual disturbance in about 10% of anovulatory women. Bromocriptine lowers prolactin levels to normal (the normal range in most laboratories being less than 20 ng/ml) and allows the ovary to get back to normal.

Side effects: The drug often causes nausea and dizziness during the first few days of treatment, but the chances of these symptoms occurring can be reduced by starting the drug at a very low dose and gradually building up to a maintenance dose of 1 to 6 tablets daily.

Dose: A 2.5 mg tablet is available; and the starting dose is usually 2.5 mg to 5 mg daily, taken at bedtime. After starting bromocriptine, prolactin levels can be tested (after at least one week of medication) to confirm that they have been brought down to normal. If the levels are still elevated, the dose will need to be increased. Once normal prolactin levels have been achieved (and some women need as much as 4 to 6 tablets a day for achieving such levels), this is then selected as the maintenance dose. The tablets must be taken daily at this dose until a pregnancy occurs, after which they should be stopped. This is expensive medication, and some pharmaceutical companies may provide it at reduced rates if the doctor requests them to do so.

Danazol

Danazol is a synthetic hormone, prescribed as one type of treatment for endometriosis. It acts by reducing the brain's production of the follicle-stimulating hormone and hence suppresses ovarian function. This is similar to an artificial menopause and results in the shrinking of not only the endometrium in the uterus (and, hence, no periods), but also hopefully the misplaced patches of endometrium outside the uterus found in patients with endometriosis, causing them to disappear.

Side effects: These are as follows: hot flushes, weight gain, acne, and hirsutism (hairiness). They can be quite troublesome, and because of them, some women have to discontinue the drug. Usually, while taking danazol, the periods will stop completely, a condition called pseudo-menopause.

Dose: The standard dose used to be 800 mg daily (4 tablets of 200 mg each). However, the side effects at this dose are considerable, and many doctors have reported good results with doses as low as 200 mg daily. The usual course of treatment is 6-9 months and the extent of the improvement in endometriosis is then reviewed. Danazol is very expensive medication!

Steroids: Dexamethasone is often used as an adjunct to ovulation induction treatment, especially in patients with hirsutism who have high levels of androgens. It helps by suppressing the production of androgens by the adrenal glands. The dose is usually a 0.5 mg tablet, taken daily at bedtime. Side effects at such a low dose are unusual.

Clomiphene

Clomiphene is the drug of first choice for inducing ovulation and is often called the doctor's "workhorse" for growing eggs. It is cheap, effective, easily available and well tolerated. It is also used for superovulating normal women to help them grow more eggs. Clomiphene is an anti-estrogen and it acts by "fooling" the pituitary into believing that estrogen levels in the body are low as a result of which the pituitary starts producing more FSH and LH – the gonadotropin hormones which, in turn, lead to stimulation of the ovaries. Only women who produce estrogen will respond to clomiphene and some doctors will test for this factor by observing if they bleed in response to progestins– a progestin challenge test.

The starting dose is one tablet (50 mg) a day for five consecutive days. The first tablet can be taken on day 2, 3, 4 or 5 of the cycle – this is usually decided by the doctor and depends on the length of the menstrual cycle. It is not enough to just take clomiphene; it is equally important to monitor the patient's response to this as well.

UNDERSTANDING YOUR MEDICINES

This is best done by serial daily vaginal ultrasound scans. The ovulation induced by clomiphene occurs about 5 to 7 days after the course of tablets is completed, that is, days 12-16 of the cycle. If ovulation fails to occur, the dose can be increased for subsequent cycles. Often human chorionic gonadotrophin (HCG) is given to trigger ovulation to mimic the woman's natural LH surge. Ultrasound and blood estrogen levels may be used to determine the best day to administer HCG. If ovulation does not occur, the patient becomes a candidate for HMG or FSH (see following paragraphs).

Usually, blood testing of progesterone levels (done 7 days after ovulation) accompanies clomiphene treatment to help identify the correct dosage needed. Clomiphene induces ovulation in approximately 70% of appropriately selected patients and has a 30% to 40% pregnancy rate.

Clomiphene increases a woman's chances of having a twin pregnancy by approximately 10%. However, the risk of having more than two babies is only 1%. Occasionally, ovarian cysts occur following clomiphene administration. These cysts usually disappear when the drug is stopped.

Side effects: Side effects can include hot flushes and mood swings early in the cycle, and depression, nausea and breast tenderness later in the cycle. Severe headaches or visual problems, though rare, are indications that the medication should be stopped.

Since clomiphene acts as an "antiestrogen", it can have an adverse effect on cervical mucus, making it thicker than usual. It is therefore important to check on sperm survival in the mucus with a postcoital or postinsemination test. If this test is consistently negative due to poor mucus, a change of medication may be advised. Alternatively, low-dose estrogens may be included in the treatment.

Long-term effects: As the drug is given only for 5 days early in the cycle, it does not have any long-term effect on future ovulation, or on hormone levels, or on pregnancy.

Misuse of clomiphene: Clomiphene can be misused because it is cheap and easy to prescribe. It is common to find patients who have been taking clomiphene for months on end, with no benefit whatsoever. Clomiphene should not be taken, unless adequate monitoring is also performed simultaneously. Clomiphene is also commonly misused as "empiric treatment", i.e., as a treatment to "enhance fertility" when the doctor cannot offer anything else.

Gonadotropins

Gonadotropin treatment can be termed "big-gun" therapy, and is usually reserved for difficult anovulatory problems. The two gonadotropin hormones, namely, the follicle-stimulating hormone (FSH) and the luteinizing hormone (LH), are produced in the pituitary gland and their secretion is controlled by a third hormone, gonadotropin-releasing hormone (GnRH), released by the hypothalamus. At the start of a new cycle, the hypothalamus begins to release GnRH. GnRH then acts on the pituitary gland to release FSH and LH. These two hormones stimulate the ovary, causing follicles to develop (as the name suggests, this is the primary action of the FSH – to stimulate follicular growth). When it is time for ovulation, a sudden burst of LH is released from the pituitary gland (the LH surge), which causes the egg to be released from the mature follicle in the ovary.

The foregoing system is a very finely tuned one, designed by Nature to ensure the release of a single mature egg every month. Such a process involves orchestrating a "symphony" of messages from the ovary, the pituitary and hypothalamus. The messages are transmitted by hormones, which act as chemical messengers in the blood stream. When the egg is ripe, the mature follicle releases an ever-increasing amount of estrogen, which is produced by the granulosa cells that line the follicle. This estrogen produced by the dominant follicle progressively increases in quantity as the egg matures, until a surge of estrogen

UNDERSTANDING YOUR MEDICINES

is released into the blood (the estrogen surge). This high level of estrogen stimulates the pituitary to release a large amount of LH hormone (the LH surge). This LH, in turn, acts on the mature follicle, causing it to rupture in order to release the mature egg. Thus, it is the mature egg which signals the brain that it is ready for release, and triggers off its own ovulation!

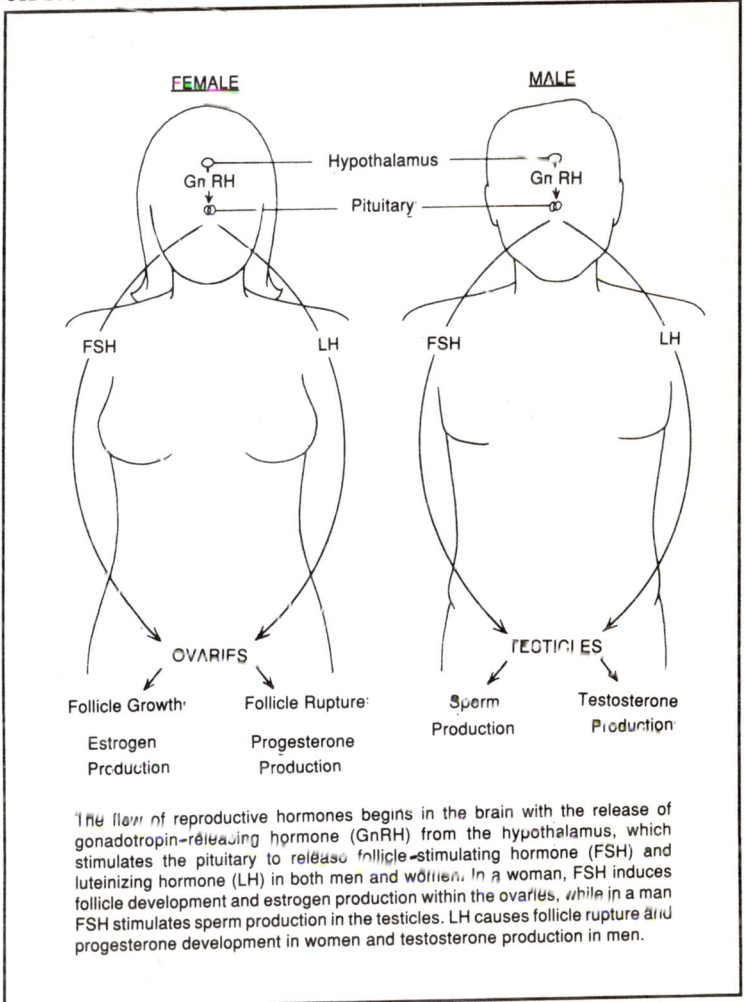

The flow of reproductive hormones begins in the brain with the release of gonadotropin-releasing hormone (GnRH) from the hypothalamus, which stimulates the pituitary to release follicle-stimulating hormone (FSH) and luteinizing hormone (LH) in both men and women. In a woman, FSH induces follicle development and estrogen production within the ovaries, while in a man FSH stimulates sperm production in the testicles. LH causes follicle rupture and progesterone development in women and testosterone production in men.

Fig. 21.1 The Flow of Reproductive Hormones

How does Nature ensure that only one egg is released every cycle? About 30-40 follicles will start growing in response to the FSH produced by the pituitary. However, only one of these follicles is destined to grow (become dominant) and rupture to release its mature egg. The others will die eventually (a process called *atresia*). The dominant follicle releases increasing amounts of estrogen as it grows bigger. This estrogen, in turn, decreases the production of FSH by the pituitary (in a negative feedback control loop), so that without high levels of FSH, the smaller follicles no longer have a stimulus to grow and they gradually die. The dominant follicle by now has become so big, that it can grow by itself, and doesn't need the additional FSH stimulation.

HMG (Human Menopausal Gonadotropin)

When the pituitary doesn't release FSH and LH or releases them in an improper balance, HMG substitutes for them and acts directly on the ovaries to stimulate the development of the follicle. HMG is a natural product containing both human FSH and LH, 75 or 150 international units (IU) of each per ampoule. This material is extracted from the urine of postmenopausal women, carefully purified and then freeze dried in sterile glass ampoules where it is sealed until use.

Very recently, biotechnology (using recombinant DNA) has been used to produce pure synthetic FSH and LH. This advance can prove to be very exciting, and may mean that these hormones will be inexpensively available in the future. However, commercial production is likely to take a few years more.

Dose: Most women need to take daily injections of HMG over a period of several days each month. The exact number of days will be determined by the physician through monitoring the response to the injections. HMG therapy usually begins on day 3 to day 5 of the menstrual cycle. If the patient is not menstruating, the injections may be started at any time. Every patient is different in her response to HMG and even the same patient may not respond in the same way from one cycle to another. Therefore, the dosage of HMG required to produce maturation of the follicle must be individualized for each patient. This factor is the key to success with these injections. It is recommended that the lowest possible dose consistent with good results be used. HMG cannot be taken orally because it is a protein and would be digested in the stomach. It is given by intramuscular injections into the buttocks or the thighs.

Side effects: Along with its intended benefits, HMG is a potent drug with the potential to cause some adverse side effects. The most common side effect with HMG relates to overstimulation of the ovary and every effort is made to avoid this by carefully monitoring the response to HMG. Mild to moderate uncomplicated ovarian enlargement, sometimes accompanied by abdominal distension and/or abdominal pain occurs in about 20% of patients treated with HMG and HCG. This complication is generally reversed without treatment within 2 to 3 weeks.

A potentially serious side effect of HMG is the hyperstimulation syndrome which is characterized by the sudden enlargement of the ovary and an accumulation of fluid in the abdomen. This fluid can also accumulate around the lungs and may cause breathing difficulties. If the ovary ruptures, blood can accumulate in the abdominal cavity, as well. The fluid imbalance can also affect blood clotting and, in rare cases, could be life threatening. Fortunately, the hyperstimulation syndrome is not common, occurring in about 1% to 3% of patients. Treatment consists of bed rest and careful monitoring of fluid levels.

Another risk arising from HMG therapy is when it becomes too successful at producing eggs, occasionally resulting in mutiple pregnancies, with their accompanying complications. Of the pregnancies following therapy with HMG, most (80%) will be single births. The multiple gestation rate is approximately 20%, the majority of which have been twins. About 5% of the total pregnancies result in three or more conceptuses. Despite careful monitoring, multiple gestations cannot be altogether avoided.

Other adverse reactions that have been reported due to HMG therapy are mild and include allergic sensitivity, pain, rash and swelling at the injection site.

Monitoring HMG Therapy

Monitoring of patients receiving HMG therapy is essential for dosage adjustment and prevention of side effects. Each woman's response is different and the dose to be prescribed needs to be adjusted carefully. The two most commonly used techniques are the determination of serum estrogen levels and ultrasound. Estrogen levels in the blood help the doctor to ascertain how well the ovaries are responding to HMG therapy and when the dose needs to be adjusted. In addition, monitoring estrogen levels helps in preventing hyperstimulation. Ultrasound allows doctors to actually observe the ovaries and determine the number of follicles which are developing and their size. Ultrasound is also used to determine when and if the ovulatory HCG injection should be given. If there are too many follicles developing, there is a greater chance of multiple births and the decision may be made to cancel the cycle by avoiding the ovulatory injection of HCG.

Studies show that about 75% of women taking HMG will ovulate. It is estimated that 20% to 42% of patients receiving HMG will become pregnant, as long as the fallopian tubes are open and the sperm count is adequate. It is mandatory that these two factors be confirmed before starting the HMG therapy!

Intercourse is advised daily or every other day beginning on the day prior to the administration of HCG.

Your doctor may want to advise you further on this point. Some doctors will perform an intrauterine insemination on the day of ovulation to increase the chances of a pregnancy.

HMG has to be imported into India, and is very expensive. It is therefore best used by infertility specialists only. The commonest use of HMG today is in IVF and GIFT programmes where it is used to stimulate several eggs to grow (superovulation).

FSH

FSH represents a more recent purified form of HMG which contains mostly FSH and negligible amounts of LH. The indications for use, administration and ovarian response are almost identical to HMG. However, as FSH contains almost no LH, it has a theoretical advantage for women with PCOS (polycystic ovarian syndrome) who characteristically have an elevated LH level. However, FSH is more expensive than HMG.

HCG

HCG is produced by the placenta during pregnancy. Because HCG is biologically very similar to LH it is used to trigger off ovulation by mimicking the natural LH surge at midcycle. HCG can be used in combination with Clomid and also HMG/FSH to induce ovulation. It is isolated and purified from the urine of pregnant women. It is available in ampoules as a sterile white powder containing 5000 IU or 10,000 IU. This powder is dissolved in a diluent and administered by IM injection.

GnRH Analogues

These drugs may be used for the treatment of endometriosis and fibroids. They work by initially stimulating and then switching off (down-regulating) the pituitary gland. These drugs are administered intranasally or by injection. They thus induce a "menopausal" state, allowing the endometriosis and fibroids to shrink, since there is no further production of estrogens.

GnRH analogues may also be used as adjunctive therapy to enhance induction of ovulation along with HMG. These analogues are prescribed when the patient's own gonadotropin secretion interferes with the administration of HMG. The patient's own (endogenous) gonadotropins (FSH and LH) are turned off by the GnRH analogues so that the physician has a clean slate to work with when administering exogenous gonadotropins to correct ovulatory disturbances.

Synthetic GnRH: GnRH stimulates the pituitary gland to secrete LH and FSH. It is used to induce ovulation in selected women with hypothalamic dysfunction. The hormone has to be given in a manner which mimics the natural secretion of LHRH, i.e., in pulses approximately 90 minutes apart. This process is carried out by means of a small pump placed under the skin of the arm or abdomen. This treatment is now given instead of HMG at certain specialist centres. Its advantage over HMG is that it produces an ovulation cycle which is similar to the natural cycle and multiple ovulation is very unusual.

Growth hormone: Some women will respond very poorly to HMG injections. They grow few or no follicles, in spite of being given large doses. In some of these "poor responders", synthetic growth hormone (HGH, human growth hormone) has been employed in order to enhance the reponse of the ovary to the HMG. This medication is very expensive, and should be used by specialists only.

Medicines Used in Male Infertility Treatments

HMG and HCG: HMG and HCG are useful in stimulating sperm production in men with hypogonadotropic hypogonadism (men with low FSH and LH levels, because of hypothalamic or pituitary malfunction), but this is a rare condition.

UNDERSTANDING YOUR MEDICINES

Treatment often takes many months to restore the sperm quality to fertile levels. Combination treatment is required – HCG stimulates testosterone production and FSH stimulates sperm production. Initially, the man takes HCG injections thrice a week for about 6 months. Such a course of injections normally causes the size of the testes to increase and the testosterone to reach normal levels. HMG injections are then added. These can be mixed with the HCG and are also given thrice a week. Once sperm production has been achieved, the HMG can be stopped; and HCG treatment continued alone. While sperm counts achieved are usually low (less than 10 million per ml), a successful pregnancy can be achieved in 50% of correctly diagnosed patients.

Unfortunately, the expensive HMG and HCG injections are often misused as empiric therapy in men with low sperm counts, with expectedly disappointing results.

Bromocriptine: As in the case of the female, bromocriptine is used to lower unusually elevated levels of prolactin.

Testosterone: Testosterone is given to suppress sperm production in the hope that when medication is stopped (usually after 5-6 months), then the sperm production will "rebound" to higher levels than the original (testosterone rebound treatment). This form of treatment is now seldom used as it may further impair fertility and is hazardous. Testosterone can also be used for the treatment of impotence or diminished libido when blood testosterone levels are low. Testosterone is available as an oily injection and is given intramuscularly, usually once a week. Oral preparations are also available now, but these are very expensive and may not be as effective

Clomiphene: Clomiphene is the most commonly prescribed medicine for infertile men. Its use is largely empirical and very controversial as the results are not predictable. This drug is usually prescribed as a 25 mg tablet, to be taken once a day, for 25 days per month, for a course of 3 to 6 months. It acts by increasing the levels of FSH and LH, which stimulate the testes to produce testosterone and sperm. The group of men who seem to benefit the most from clomiphene have low sperm counts, with low or low-normal gonadotropin levels. However, while clomiphene may increase sperm counts in selected men, it hasn't been proven effective in increasing pregnancy rates.

Antibiotics: Just as in the female, antibiotics can resolve a chronic infection in the reproductive tract in the male. Often no specific organism is isolated but improvement in the numbers of normal sperm as well as the reduction in white cells in semen can be seen in some men following several weeks of antibiotic treatment.

Vitamins: No supportive evidence exists at present that vitamins are helpful in improving sperm production, but, sometimes, they are worth a try.

Ayurvedic Treatment and Other Magic Potions

Everyone seems to have a "magic potion" to cure low sperm counts – the trouble is that no one has ever proven that anything works! Take all such claims with a liberal pinch of salt.

The problem with the medical treatment of a low sperm count is that for most patients it simply doesn't work. The very fact that there are so many ways of "treating" a low sperm count itself suggests that there is no effective method available. This is the sad state of affairs today and much needs to be learnt about the causes of low sperm production before we can find effective methods of treating this disorder.

Patients, nevertheless, want treatment; so there is pressure on the doctor to prescribe, even if he knows the therapy may not be helpful. (The logic is : "Anyway it can't hurt".) The doctor also remembers the anecdotal successes (those who come back for follow-up, while the others desert the doctor and are lost to follow-up). After all, what else is there to do? This is why patients with low sperm counts are subjected to every treatment imaginable – with little rational basis – Vitamin E, Vitamin C, high-protein diets, homoeopathic pills, ayurvedic *churans* and ice-cold baths. However, this attitude can be positively harmful. It wastes time, during which the wife gets older, and her fertility potential decreases. Patients are unhappy when there is no improvement in the sperm count and lose confidence in doctors. It also stops the patient from exploring effective modes of alternative therapy, such as IVF and GIFT. Today empiric therapy should be criticized unless it is used as a short-term therapeutic trial with a clearly defined end-point.

A word of warning: Medical treatment for male infertility does not have a high success rate and has unpleasant side effects, so don't go in for it unless your doctor explains his rationale. The treatment is best considered "experimental" and can be tried as a therapeutic trial. Make sure, however, that semen is examined for improvement after three months and then decide whether you want to press on regardless.

It is worth emphasizing how small the list for male infertility treatment is, especially as compared to female treatment. This simply reflects our ignorance about male infertility – we know very little about what causes it, and our knowledge about how to treat it is even more pitiable!

22

Artificial Insemination by the Husband's Sperm

SOMETIMES MOTHER NATURE NEEDS HELP to start a pregnancy, and the doctor can provide such help by giving the sperm a "piggyback ride" through a fine tube into the body. This procedure is called *artificial insemination*, and, effectively, the doctor is giving Nature a helping hand by increasing the chances of the egg and sperm meeting.

Artificial insemination by husband (AIH) is useful in the following cases:

1. The woman has a cervical mucus problem. For example, the mucus may be scanty or hostile to the sperm. With an intrauterine insemination (IUI), the sperm can bypass her cervix and enter the uterine cavity directly.
2. The man has antibodies to his own sperm. The "good" sperm which have not been affected by the antibodies are separated in the laboratory and used for IUI.
3. If the man cannot ejaculate into his partner's vagina. This situation arises because of psychological problems such as impotence (inability to get and maintain an erection) and vaginismus

(an involuntary spasm of the vaginal muscles so that vaginal penetration is not possible); or because of anatomic problems of the penis, such as uncorrected hypospadias; or if the man is paraplegic.

4. The man suffers from retrograde ejaculation in which the semen goes backward into the bladder instead of coming out of the penis.
5. For unexplained infertility, since the technique of IUI increases the chances of the eggs and sperm meeting.
6. As an inexpensive alternative to GIFT, IUI is a reasonable first choice (especially for younger couples) since it is so much cheaper and less intrusive.
7. If the husband is away from the wife for long stretches of time (for example, husbands who work on ships or work abroad), his sperm can be frozen and stored in a sperm bank and used to inseminate his wife even in his absence.
8. For male factor infertility, though this is a controversial area, especially for the common problem of oligospermia (a low sperm count). What is the rationale behind using IUI for treating this problem? Remember that infertility is a problem of the couple's, not just the oligospermic male's. Whether a given couple will conceive or not depends on the sum of their fertility potentials. Therefore, the fertility potential of the wife is improved by superovulating her, so that instead of producing just one egg per cycle, she produces 2-4 eggs per cycle. In addition, the husband's sperm are processed in the laboratory, and the best sperm are used for IUI. This increases the chances of the best sperm being able to reach and fertilize the egg.

Methods for Performing AIH

There are various methods of performing AIH. The crudest and simplest technique involves simply injecting the entire semen sample into the vagina by a syringe. However, this is a waste of time if used for treating an infertility problem; after all, why go to a doctor to do something which you can do for yourself at home? Remember, a syringe is no better than a penis. It is only useful if the reason for doing AIH is the inability of the husband to ejaculate in the vagina. However, a number of doctors still use it as they do not have anything better to offer.

A refinement of the aforementioned technique is that of using a split ejaculate. The first squirt of semen which gushes forth during ejaculation is the richest in sperm. This is because the sperm surf on the wave of the seminal fluid which carries them forward to the outside world. The man masturbates into a two-part container, so that the first part of the ejaculate goes into one container, while the rest goes into another. This is not as difficult as it sounds, and the procedure becomes easier with practice! The first container is saved and the contents used for artificial insemination. This method is suitable for a small proportion of cases (for example, for the uncommon problem of a large volume of semen, which dilutes the sperm; or where laboratory facilities for sperm processing are not available).

Intrauterine Insemination (IUI)

In the IUI method, the sperm are removed from the seminal fluid by processing the semen in the laboratory and then they are injected directly into the uterine cavity. It is not advisable to inject the semen directly into the uterus, as the semen contains chemicals (prostaglandins) and pus cells which can cause severe cramping and even tubal infection.

Timing

Timing the IUI is very important. It must be done during the "fertile" period when the egg is present in the fallopian tube. Pinpointing the time of ovulation accurately using either vaginal ultrasound or ovulation test kits is crucial. A good clinic should provide this as a 7-day week service, since there is a 1 in 7 chance that ovulation will occur on a Sunday - eggs don't take a holiday! Often the wife's fertility potential is also simultaneously increased by drugs so that she produces more than one egg per cycle (superovulation) to increase the chances of conception.

The IUI is done either when ovulation is imminent or just after. The husband masturbates into a clean jar, preferably in the laboratory or clinic itself, after at least three days of sexual abstinence in order to get optimal sperm counts. The best sperm are separated from the rest of the seminal fluid by special laboratory processing techniques. This separation takes about 1 to 2 hours. The actual insemination procedure is simple and takes only a few minutes to perform. It is not painful, though it can be uncomfortable. The wife lies on an examining table, and a speculum is placed in the vagina. The doctor puts the sperm through a thin plastic tube (catheter) through the cervix into the uterus. There may be a bit of uterine cramping at this time; and some discomfort for about 12 to 24 hours. No special bed rest is required after this procedure, as the sperm cannot "fall out" of the uterine cavity. Some doctors may repeat the insemination after 24 hours.

Sperm Processing

Sperm processing allows the doctor to concentrate the actively motile sperm into a small volume of culture fluid Sperm do not remain alive in the culture medium for very long unless maintained at just the right conditions; hence, a prompt insemination after sperm processing is vital. This is why processing should preferably be done in the clinic itself, so that time is not wasted in transporting the sperm after the wash.

Laboratory Techniques

There are different methods of processing the sperm, and all of them require special laboratory expertise.

1. The simplest method is that of washing the semen with a culture medium (by centrifuging it and collecting the pellet), but this is a poor technique and is not recommended.

2. The swim-up method uses a layering technique, in which a special culture medium is placed above the semen in a test tube. The good quality sperm will swim up into the culture medium, and after 45 to 60 minutes, this medium (with the motile sperm) is removed and injected into the uterine cavity.

3. The more sophisticated methods today use a Percoll column. This column allows one to separate the good quality sperm from the immotile sperm, the pus cells and the seminal plasma, because these are lighter than the motile sperm. It provides the best recovery of motile sperm and is the standard technique in use today, especially for poor quality sperm samples.

Recent Advances

Of late, doctors have tried adding various chemicals to the washed sperm to try to improve their motility, so as to increase the chances of their reaching their goal. These chemicals include caffeine and pentoxyfylline and they may be helpful to some patients.

During IUI, sperm are injected into the uterine cavity in the hope that they will then swim up from here into the fallopian tubes where they can fertilize the egg. But then, why not inject the sperm directly into the fallopian tubes where the egg is present? This feat was technically difficult to accomplish in the past, because the fallopian tubes are so thin. Today, with specially designed catheters (Jansen-Anderson catheter sets), it is possible to carry out this procedure in the doctor's clinic. Thus, the processed sperm can be injected directly into the tubes under ultrasound guidance, without anesthesia or surgery! This is an intratubal insemination – also known as a SIFT (sperm intrafallopian transfer).

Psychological Issues

Men may feel a loss of self-esteem because they think that they need a doctor's help to do what a "normal man" should have been able to do by himself. They also feel guilty about having to subject their wife to the pain and intrusion of insemination. Women may feel anger towards their husbands for having the fertility problem. The insemination may also make patients feel that someone has "intruded" into their sex life and this may affect their intimacy.

Success Rate of AIH

The success rate of AIH depends upon several factors. First of all, the cause of the infertility problem is important. For example, men with normal sperm counts, who are unable to have intercourse, have a much higher chance of success than patients who are undergoing AIH for poor sperm counts. In addition, female factors play an important role. If the female is more than 35, the chance of a successful pregnancy is significantly decreased. Generally, the chance of conceiving in one cycle is about 10-15%, and the cumulative conception rate is about 60% over 5-6 treatment cycles. (Remember, Nature's efficiency for producing a baby in one month is only about 15% to 25%.) However, if AIH is going to prove effective for a couple, it usually does so within 6 treatment cycles. If a pregnancy has not resulted in this time, the chances of

AIH working for them are very remote, and they should stop persisting with this procedure and explore other possibilites. However, one should start AIH with the expectation that it may take about 6 treatment cycles.

The Cost Factor

The cost of performing AIH varies from clinic to clinic, but is about Rs 1000 to Rs 3000 for the entire treatment cycle. Of course, if gonadotropin injections are used for superovulation, the treatment then becomes much more expensive, and can go up to as much as Rs 10,000 for one month's treatment.

AIH is a simple, inexpensive, effective form of therapy, and can usually be tried first, before going on to more expensive and invasive options. However, it can be very stressful and close cooperation between the husband and wife (and the doctor!) is essential!

23

Test Tube Babies -- IVF and GIFT

THE BIRTH OF LOUISE BROWN THROUGH *in vitro* fertilization (IVF) in 1978 dramatically increased awareness of clinical alternatives for the infertile couple. Today, new techniques for assisted reproduction are evolving rapidly.

This chapter will help you understand assisted reproductive technologies such as IVF and gamete intrafallopian transfer (GIFT) that have become accepted medical treatments for infertility. For many couples who have exhausted traditional clinical and surgical treatments for infertility, these new technologies may offer the best hope for pregnancy. Through these procedures, women with otherwise untreatable infertility problems have given birth to healthy babies.

IVF

IVF is a method of assisted reproduction in which the man's sperm and the woman's egg are combined in a laboratory dish, where fertilization occurs. The resulting embryo is transferred to the woman's uterus. The basic steps in an IVF treatment cycle are ovulation enhancement (stimulating the development of more than one egg in a cycle), egg harvest, fertilization, embryo culture, and embryo transfer.

IVF can be a reasonable treatment choice for couples with various types of infertility. Initially, it was only used when the woman had blocked, damaged, or absent fallopian tubes (tubal factor infertility). IVF is now also used to circumvent infertility caused by endometriosis, immunological problems, unexplained infertility, and male factor infertility.

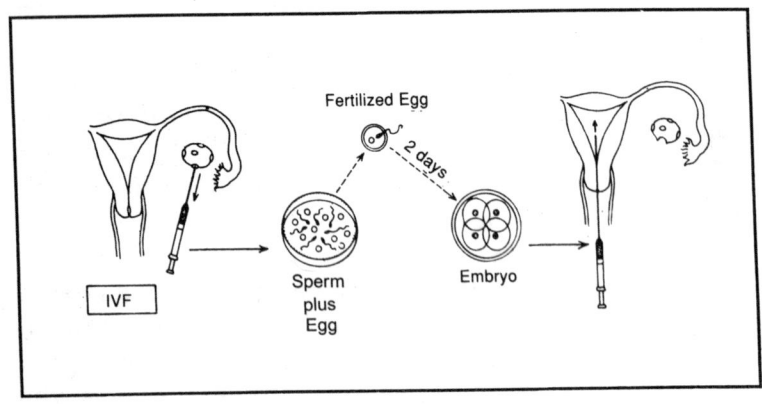

Fig. 23.1   IVF

Tests Prior to IVF

First, a *sperm survival test* is carried out. This is a "trial" sperm wash, using exactly the same method as will be actually used in IVF, to assess whether an adequate number of sperm can be recovered in order to perform IVF. This test will also help the laboratory to decide which method of sperm processing should be used during IVF.

A useful test for older women, in order to assess their suitability for IVF, may be a blood test called a *clomiphene stimulated FSH level*, which gives a rough idea of how many eggs will be grown as a result of superovulation. If the level is very high, this suggests early ovarian failure, and it may be a better idea to consider donor eggs.

Many clinics may do a hysteroscopy, in order to assess that the uterine cavity is totally normal. They may also do a "dummy" embryo transfer to make sure there are no technical problems with this procedure. Some clinics also do a cervical swab test, to rule out the presence of infection in the cervix.

Blood tests which may be done include tests for immunity to rubella, and tests for Hepatitis B, and AIDS.

Patients who stand a very poor chance of success with IVF include the following:

- Older women, whose ovaries are failing. However, there is no upper age limit at which IVF should not be done, and, in fact, for older women, it might represent their only chance of success. It's not really the age of the woman which is the limiting factor; it's the quality of her eggs.
- Men whose sperm count is very low. Again, IVF may be the only option these men have to father their own biological child; and, therefore, there is no "magic" number of sperm which a man must have before considering IVF for him.
- Women with a damaged uterus (for example, because of healed tuberculosis) because the chance of successful implantation of the embryo in the uterus becomes very poor.

It is also not advisable to go in for IVF treatment without trying simpler treatment options first. IVF is a complex procedure involving considerable personal and financial commitment, so other treatments are usually recommended first.

The Basic Steps of IVF

Superovulation or Ovulation Enhancement

During superovulation, drugs are used to induce the patient's ovaries to grow several mature eggs rather than the single egg that normally develops each month. This is done because the chances of pregnancy become higher if more than one egg is fertilized and transferred to the uterus during a treatment cycle. Depending on the programme and the patient, the drug type and the dosage vary. Most often, the drugs are given over a period of seven to ten days. Drugs currently in use include: clomiphene citrate, human menopausal gonadotropin (HMG), follicle-stimulating hormone (FSH), human chorionic gonadotropin (HCG), human growth hormone (HGH) and gonodotropin-releasing hormone (GnRH) analogue. These drugs may be used alone or in combination with others.

Timing is crucial during an IVF treatment cycle. The doctor not only must know what is happening in the woman's ovaries but also when it happens. To monitor the development of ovarian follicles the ovaries are scanned frequently with ultrasound. Blood samples may be drawn to measure the serum levels of estrogen and luteinizing hormone (LH).

By interpreting the results of ultrasound and blood tests, the doctor determines the best time to harvest or remove the eggs. When the follicles are mature the doctor prescribes an injection of human chorionic gonadotropin (HCG). The use of HCG allows the doctor to control when ovulation will actually take place, usually about 36 hours after the HCG injection. This control allows the IVF team to be prepared to harvest eggs just before that time. The HCG simulates the woman's natural LH surge, which normally triggers off ovulation.

Ovulation may occur naturally during some treatment cycles, despite the use of these drugs and this is called "spontaneous ovulation". When this occurs, the eggs may be lost in the pelvic cavity, and the next step in the treatment cycle must be cancelled. In some cases, however, a spontaneous LH surge can be detected by blood and urine tests before the eggs are released. Ultrasound can confirm that the eggs are still in their follicles. If they are, the doctor may decide to harvest the eggs earlier than originally scheduled.

With older forms of superovulation regimes using clomiphene and HMG, the treatment cycle was cancelled in roughly one quarter of the IVF cycles. The women whose cycles were cancelled either had responded poorly to drugs used for ovulation enhancement or had premature, spontaneously occurring LH surges with resulting premature ovulation. Cancellation rates as low as 5% have been achieved in some IVF programmes using the newer GnRH analogues in combination with gonadotropins during ovulation enhancement. Treatment with the analogues prevents the release of FSH and LH from the pituitary gland during treatment ("down regulation") and thereby prevents premature ovulation. Such a situation, therefore, gives the doctor much better control over the superovulation phase.

Egg Harvest

Egg harvest is usually accomplished today by ultrasound-guided aspiration. This procedure is a minor surgical one that can be done even under intravenous sedation. The ultrasound probe is inserted through the vagina. The probe emits high-frequency sound waves which are translated into images of the pelvic organs and displayed on a monitor. When a mature follicle is identified, the specialist guides a needle through the vagina and into the follicle. The follicular fluid containing the egg is then sucked out through the needle into a test tube.

The older method of performing egg retrieval involved a laparoscopy. The eggs and follicular fluid were aspirated under direct vision. However, this method is rarely used today, because the vaginal ultrasound-guided method is much quicker, easier and safer.

Insemination, Fertilization and Embryo Culture

The aspirated follicular fluid is next examined in the laboratory and the eggs identified and graded for maturity.

The maturity of an egg determines when the sperm should be added to it (insemination). Insemination can be done at three points of time: immediately upon harvest; after several hours or on the following day.

On the day the eggs are harvested, the husband provides a semen sample. The sperm are separated from the seminal plasma in a process known as "washing the sperm". The washed sperm are used to inseminate the eggs.

A defined number of sperm is placed with each egg in a separate dish containing the IVF culture medium. The dishes are placed in an incubator with a controlled temperature that is the same as the woman's body, i.e., 37°C.

It takes about 18 hours for fertilization to be completed, and about 12 hours later, the fertilized cell or embryo divides into two cells. The embryo may divide several times while in the incubator. After 48 hours, when embryos usually consist of two to four cells each, they are ready to be placed in the woman's uterus. This procedure is known as "embryo transfer".

Embryo Transfer

Embryo transfer is most often done in a clinic or hospital on an outpatient basis. No anesthesia is used, although some women may wish to have a mild sedative. The patient lies on a table or bed, usually with her feet in stirrups. Some clinics perform the transfer with the patient in the knee-chest position. Using a vaginal speculum, the doctor exposes the cervix. One or more embryos suspended in a drop of culture medium are drawn into a transfer catheter, a long, thin sterile tube with a syringe at one end. Gently, the doctor guides the tip of the loaded catheter through the cervix and deposits the fluid into the uterine cavity. One or more embryos may be transferred during this procedure. The entire transfer procedure usually takes between 10 and 20 minutes. Some doctors recommend bed rest after the embryo transfer. After the transfer, some clinics also provide "luteal phase support" through progesterone injections, progesterone suppositories, or HCG injections.

The embryo transfer completes the medical treatment in the IVF cycle. However, this is the stage when the hardest part of an IVF cycle for the patient starts – the agony and suspense of waiting to find out whether or not a pregnancy has occurred. This can be determined by blood HCG tests only 10 to 14 days after the transfer.

Thus, there are numerous stages to every IVF treatment cycle, each of which must be reached and completed before moving on to the next stage:

- treatment should be available when you want it;
- more than one egg should develop;
- blood hormone levels should rise sufficiently;
- eggs should mature;
- ovulation should not occur before the eggs can be collected;
- eggs must be retrieved during the "pick-up";
- sperm must fertilize at least one egg;
- fertilized eggs must divide and grow healthily ... and all this so that...
- the embryos might get implanted in the uterus.

Think of the process as a series of hurdles, all of which have to be cleared.

The Cost of IVF

The cost of a single IVF treatment cycle varies widely from approximately Rs 30,000 to more than Rs 75,000 depending on the programme and the items included in the fee. It is important to get an itemized listing from the selected programme of what costs have been included in the treatment cycle. Other expenses to be aware of include time missed from work, and travel and lodging expenses.

The number of treatment cycles needed to achieve pregnancy will, of course, determine the final cost.

Alternatives

A reduction in cost may be obtained by using the "natural cycle" for IVF. This procedure does not employ ovulation enhancement; therefore, the additional expense on the injections used for superovulation is eliminated. However, only one egg is usually obtained, and the pregnancy rate per cycle is therefore less for this method.

Embryo Freezing

Since most IVF programmes superovulate patients to grow many eggs, there are often many embryos. Since the risk of multiple pregnancies increases with the number of embryos transferred (and, in fact, the law in the UK prohibits the transfer of more than three embryos to reduce this risk), many patients are left with spare or supernumerary embryos. These can be discarded or else used for research. It is now also possible to freeze these embryos and store them in liquid nitrogen. This is an expensive procedure and about half the embryos die as a result of the freezing. However, these stored embryos can then be used later for the same patient so that she can have another embryo transfer cycle done without having to go through superovulation and egg harvest. Moreover, since this embryo transfer can be done in a "natural" cycle (when she is not taking any hormone medications) some doctors believe the receptivity of the uterus to the embryos would be better. For women with irregular menstrual cycles, frozen embryo transfer can also be done in a "simulated natural cycle", in which the endometrium is primed to maximize its receptivity to the embryos by using exogenous estrogens and progesterone.

Once stored, embryos can be used by the couple during a later treatment cycle, donated to another couple or removed from storage. These options should only be undertaken after considerable discussion and written consent from the parties concerned.

GIFT

GIFT stands for *gamete intrafallopian transfer*. A gamete is a male or female sex cell – a sperm or an egg. During GIFT, sperm and eggs are mixed and injected into one or both fallopian tubes. After the gametes have been transferred, fertilization can take place in the fallopian tube as it does in natural, unassisted reproduction. Once fertilized, the embryo travels to the uterus by natural processes.

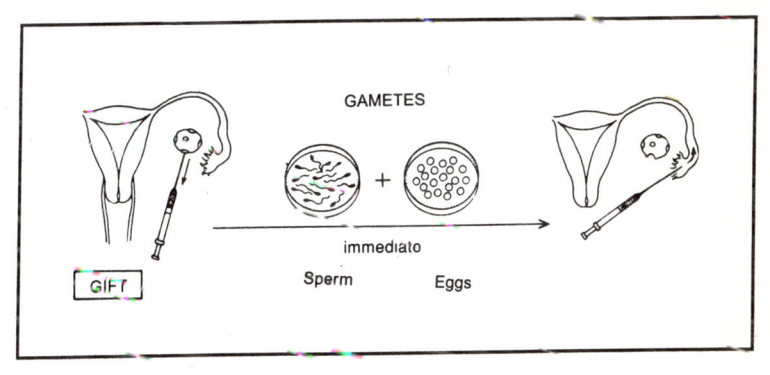

Fig. 23.2   GIFT

As in IVF, a GIFT treatment cycle begins with ovulation enhancement which is followed by egg harvest, usually by means of laparoscopy. But the similarity to IVF ends here. In IVF, an embryo is transferred. In GIFT, only gametes are transferred.

Only patients who have at least one normal, healthy fallopian tube are candidates for GIFT. Such patients include women who have unexplained infertility or mild endometriosis, and couples whose infertility results from male, cervical, or immunological factors. Some doctors recommend that couples with male factor infertility proceed with GIFT only if it has been proven that the man's sperm can fertilize the woman's egg either by *in vitro* fertilization or by past pregnancies.

The Basic Steps of GIFT

The basic steps of GIFT are ovulation enhancement, egg harvest, insemination, and gamete transfer. The eggs are usually harvested during laparoscopy. During this same laparoscopy procedure, which takes about an hour, eggs are mixed with sperm and the gametes are transferred.

Insemination

The harvested eggs are examined under the microscope and graded for maturity. The selected eggs are placed in individual dishes and combined with sperm (insemination). The sperm are prepared in advance in the same manner as for IVF. Many programmes load eggs and sperm individually into a catheter and inject them into one or both of the fallopian tubes.

Gamete Transfer

The sperm-egg mixture is loaded into a specially designed catheter. This mixture is then directed into the fallopian tube(s) through their fimbrial opening while looking through the laparoscope. Up to four eggs and sperm may be injected into one or both tubes. Gametes will be transferred only if the fallopian tubes appear healthy. If the surgeon determines that the tubes are unhealthy, IVF should be attempted instead. For this reason, GIFT should be undertaken only at facilities that have the capability to perform IVF also.

Pregnancy Rates

Specialists generally agree that pregnancy rates are higher for GIFT than for IVF; in fact, GIFT is about twice as successful as IVF. In part, this higher pregnancy rate may be due to the type of patient accepted into GIFT programmes. It may also be because the *in vivo* tubal environment is more "physiologic" for the gametes and embryo than the *in vitro* environment.

The advantages of the GIFT technique are:

- The fallopian tube acts as the laboratory.
- The embryo will reach the uterus at a later stage in its development, as in the case of normal conception.
- The procedure is considered morally acceptable to some religious groups, which object to IVF, as conception occurs within the human body.
- The endometrium will also be more receptive to the embryo because of the greater time the embryo takes to reach the uterus.

GIFT and IVF Compared

There are several differences between GIFT and IVF. The most important one is that GIFT requires healthy fallopian tubes, whereas IVF is appropriate treatment for women with tubal disease, or even those with no fallopian tubes at all. At present, GIFT requires laparoscopy for transfer. An IVF treatment cycle can be complete without laparoscopy.

In the case of GIFT, fertilization occurs unobserved inside the body, whereas in IVF, fertilization takes place in a laboratory dish and can be confirmed visually under a microscope. Visual confirmation of fertilization is especially important in cases of male factor infertility or unexplained infertility. [To obtain visual confirmation and still have the greater chance of pregnancy afforded by GIFT, one of the variations of GIFT described later (ZIFT, PROST or TET) may be used, to give the patient the benefit of combining the advantages of both the procedures.]

Vaginal GIFT

A major disadvantage with conventional GIFT is that a surgical procedure, namely, laparoscopy, is needed to transfer the eggs and sperm into the fallopian tube. Recently, a non-surgical method has been described by Dr Robert Jansen and Dr John Anderson from Sydney, Australia, in which the gametes can be transferred into the fallopian tubes through the vagina and cervix under ultrasound guidance. This requires a special set of catheters which allow the doctor to enter the uterine ends of the fallopian tubes through the cervix. Once the catheters have been accurately positioned – and ultrasound can help in this procedure – the gametes are injected into the tubes. Since this method does not involve surgery, the benefits to the patient are obvious – less expense, no hospitalization, no scar and no anesthesia. However, the technique does require much more technical expertise and is still being investigated more thoroughly. Also, the pregnancy rates with the method are less than those with conventional laparoscopic GIFT.

The Cost of GIFT

The cost of a GIFT treatment cycle varies from one programme to another, falling within the same basic range of Rs 30,000 to Rs 75,000 plus, which is typical for IVF.

Variations of GIFT

Variations of GIFT include procedures with names like ZIFT, PROST, and TET – an alphabetic potpourri !

ZIFT, i.e., zygote intrafallopian transfer, is also called PROST, which stands for pronuclear stage transfer. When a sperm penetrates an egg, the sperm introduces its nuclear material into the egg. Approximately 14 hours after penetration, two distinct pronuclei, one from the sperm and one from the egg, are visible under the microscope. Pronuclei are taken as indicators that fertilization has occurred. The fertilized egg before cell division begins is also called a "zygote". During ZIFT, eggs are removed by transvaginal aspiration and fertilized in a laboratory dish. The next day, when the fertilized eggs have reached the pronuclear stage, the embryos are transferred to the fallopian tubes during laparoscopy.

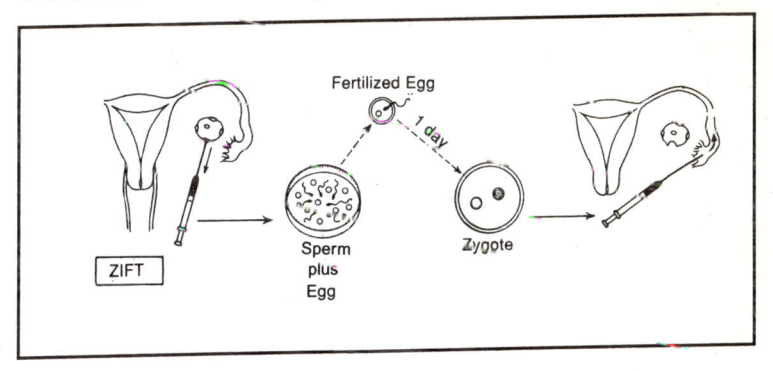

Fig. 23.3   ZIFT

Approximately 24 hours after a fertilized egg reaches the pronuclear stage, it divides for the first time and becomes a two-cell embryo. This cell division is called "cleavage". It is at this stage or later that TET (tubal embryo transfer) may be attempted. The fertilized and dividing eggs (early cleavage stage embryos) are transferred to the fallopian tube during laparoscopy.

PROST, ZIFT and TET differ from GIFT in that fertilization takes place in a laboratory dish instead of the fallopian tube. Moreover, they differ from IVF in that the fertilized egg is transferred to the fallopian tube instead of to the uterus. They offer the best of both IVF and GIFT, namely, documentation of fertilization *in vitro* and also higher pregnancy rates because of tubal transfer. However, the cost of ZIFT, PROST, or TET is usually greater than that of IVF or GIFT.

Success Rates – Making Sense of the Figures

The most important question most patients ask about IVF and GIFT is: What are the chances of achieving pregnancy? This is a difficult question to answer, since there are so many variables involved. Chances of success depend upon:

- The wife's age – chances decline with increasing age, precipitously so over the age of 40.
- The reason for the IVF/GIFT – chances of pregnancy decline when IVF is done for male factor infertility.
- The quality of the IVF clinic and its services.
- The number of embryos/eggs transferred.
- The superovulation regime used.

Of course, there are some variables about which nothing can be done, such as the wife's age. But other variables can be controlled to try to maximize chances of a pregnancy!

Pregnancy rates are related directly to how many embryos are transferred. For example, when three embryos are transferred, the chance of pregnancy is 20% in that cycle. The number of embryos transferred needs also to be balanced against the risk of multiple pregnancy, which naturally increases with more embryos. With this fact in mind, the Fertility Society of Australia recommends that no more than three embryos be transferred during any treatment cycle.

Studies done the world over show that the average pregnancy rate per cycle for IVF is about 15% for most patients, and about 30% for GIFT. How can a patient interpret this figure? For example, let us consider a 30-year-old patient with irreparable tubal damage who goes through one IVF cycle. She can look at the pregnancy rate figure of 15% in two ways. A success rate of 15% means there is an 85% chance she will not get pregnant. On the other hand, if she does not go in for any treatment, her chance of getting pregnant is zero. The IVF cycle has increased this to 15% – no one can do any better than this today! Of course, for the couple who gets a baby, it's a 100% baby, and for the one who fails, it's 0%. For the individual patient, it's really not a question of statistics!

IVF and GIFT treatment should not be considered to be a single shot affair. Patients should plan (mentally at least!) to go through at least three to four cycles to give themselves a fair chance of getting pregnant. With four treatment cycles, the chance of getting pregnant (the cumulative conception rate) is about 50%. What this means is that even though the chance of getting pregnant in a single cycle may never be more than 20%, over a period of four treatment cycles, the chances increase to 50% because the success rate is cumulative. Thus, let us assume the pregnancy rate for IVF at a clinic is 20%. If 10 patients start an IVF cycle, two will get pregnant, leaving eight patients. If these eight patients go through another IVF cycle, another 20% (1.6 patients – so let's say another one) will conceive. If the remaining seven go through another cycle, one more will get pregnant and at the end of the fourth cycle, one more will conceive, so that of the 10 patients who started, five would have become pregnant in four attempts. This is because the chances of getting pregnant in the next IVF cycle do not decrease just because a pregnancy has not occurred in the previous cycle, so the best bet would be to keep on trying. Of course, one has to set a limit somewhere, and the decision when to stop is something which only the couple can make for themselves. After more than six failed IVF cycles, the chance for a pregnancy with IVF does decline.

Games IVF Clinics Play with Pregnancy Rates

Of course, some clinics have achieved much better pregnancy rates than others. Nevertheless, many clinics will quote inflated rates – and this can mislead patients!

Unfortunately, in India there is no central registry or monitoring of IVF clinics, so that you pretty much have to trust what the doctor tells you. In many countries in the West, the law mandates that IVF clinics provide their pregnancy rates to a central authority, thus ensuring that IVF clinics maintain high standards and quality control. This regulation can be very helpful for patients.

Different programmes define success in different ways. To most couples, success means the birth of a baby, not just a pregnancy, so that what needs to be determined is the "take-home baby rate". Some clinics quote success rates as pregnancy rates, and these figures can be considerably higher than the live birth rate, depending upon how a pregnancy is defined. Thus, some programmes define pregnancy when the pregnancy test is positive; others define pregnancy as a fetus seen on ultrasound.

So-called biochemical pregnancies are also fairly common after IVF. These are pregnancies confirmed by blood and urine tests but in which the embryo does not develop beyond the earliest stage. No gestational sac or fetus is seen on ultrasound examination. Counting biochemical pregnancies will, of course, inflate the pregnancy rate.

Most programmes today express their pregnancy rate as clinical pregnancies per treatment cycle. A clinical pregnancy is one with an increasing level of the pregnancy hormone, HCG, and the presence of a gestational sac detected by ultrasound. Even if a clinical pregnancy is established, there is still a chance of miscarriage or ectopic pregnancy.

Newer Procedures

IVF technology is improving by leaps and bounds and many exciting advances have taken place recently. Many of these are now available in India, and these include the following.

Assisted Fertilization

One of the major problems with IVF today is the low pregnancy rate after successful embryo transfer. The reason why such few embryos get implanted successfully (only one out of 10 embryos will become a baby) is one of the things we do not really understand today. Dr Jacques Cohen from New York believes this is because the surrounding shell of the embryo (called the zona pellucida) hardens when it is cultured in the laboratory. Dr Cohen and associates therefore use embryo surgery (called zona drilling) to soften the shell of the embryo, and they believe this helps in increasing pregnancy rates by improving implantation rates, since embryo hatching is facilitated.

Embryo surgery has also been used for embryo biopsy, in which single cells are removed from the developing embryo, in order to make sure that the embryos are healthy and have no genetic disease.

Other scientists feel that the reason for the poor implantation can be attributed to the poor quality of the embryo cultured *in vitro*. They have, therefore, tried to improve embryo quality in the laboratory by trying to provide it with more natural ("physiological") culture conditions. This is done by a method called "co-culture" in which the embryo is cultured along with "feeder cells" in the culture dish. These cells provide the embryo with the extra nourishment needed for better growth. Better pregnancy rates are claimed with co-cultured embryos as compared to embryos grown under traditional IVF conditions.

A dramatic advance with regard to IVF for severe male factor infertility has been the development of the technique of microinjection in recent years. In this method, a single sperm is injected directly into the egg by the scientist under microscopic control. Such an injection can be done with specially prepared fine glass microneedles and even with laser beams! This technique truly represents the next generation of IVF technology!

Some people might question whether all the aforementioned advances are relevant to Indian conditions. While these technological refinements are very exciting, IVF clinics in India should also focus on simplifying IVF technology, so that it can be made more affordable for the average Indian couple. Advances which have helped to simplify IVF and make it more easily available include the following.

Intravaginal culture: This is a technique for IVF, which provides the same rate of fertilization that conventional IVF does, at a fraction of the cost. In this method, which was first described by Dr Claude Ranoux of France in 1984, the eggs and sperm are placed in a sterile vial which is then sealed and placed in the woman's vagina. Thus, the woman acts like her own incubator, since she keeps her eggs and embryos at body temperature. Since expensive laboratory equipment is not needed, this method is much cheaper, and is as effective as conventional IVF!

Natural cycle IVF: Natural cycle IVF is much less expensive than conventional IVF because it does away with the high expense of gonadotropin injections used for superovulation. In this method, the single egg which the woman grows in her unstimulated ovulatory cycle is used for IVF. While the pregnancy rate is lower, the expense (and the stress of IVF) is much less!

Transport IVF: Transport IVF is a recent innovation pioneered by scientists in the Netherlands and also by Dr Charles Kingsland of the UK. In this method, the egg retrieval is performed by the gynecologist in his own clinic or hospital and the eggs (in the follicular fluid) are then transported to a central IVF laboratory by the husband in a portable incubator. Insemination, fertilization and embryo transfer take place in the central laboratory. This method has the following plus points: (i) it allows gynecologists to take an active part in their patients' treatment; (ii) it ensures high quality, since all laboratory procedures are performed in a central laboratory; and (iii) it minimizes the inconvenience caused to the patient (since superovulation and egg retrieval are done by the local gynecologist, the number of visits the patient has to make to the IVF centre is minimized).

Donor Sperm and Eggs

Couples who are unable to produce sperm or eggs can undergo IVF and GIFT with the use of donor sperm or eggs.

For IVF, cryopreserved donor sperm are processed in the same way as fresh sperm. In some cases of female infertility, fertilization may be attempted first with the husband's sperm, and if this fails, donor sperm may be used in a second attempt. Alternatively, if several eggs are aspirated, some may be inseminated with the partner's sperm and some with donor sperm.

Donor eggs can be used in GIFT or IVF for women who are unable to grow eggs (ovarian failure), but who do have a healthy uterus. For GIFT, the woman must also have at least one functional fallopian tube. In GIFT, the donor's eggs are mixed with sperm from the husband. This mixture is injected into the patient's fallopian tubes, while hormone supplements prepare the uterus and aid in the initiation of pregnancy. For IVF, embryos resulting from the fertilization of donor eggs and the husband's sperm are placed directly inside the patient's uterus.

A couple may also choose to use donor eggs if the woman is suffering from a genetic disease that could be passed on to a child. Donor eggs can also be used in some cases of long-standing infertility when other procedures have failed — for example, women with many previous unsuccessful IVF cycles. The use of egg donation is now becoming increasingly common, as older women are seeking infertility treatment. Since the chance of a pregnancy in the older woman depends directly upon the quality of her eggs, many older women opt to use donor eggs from younger women – which increases their pregnancy rates dramatically. Such a development also creates headline news; for example, when a menopausal woman has given birth with donor eggs. In rare cases, when both the man and woman are infertile, donor sperm and donor eggs have been used together.

Unfortunately, it is still not possible to freeze and store eggs – they are too fragile! This is why fresh eggs need to be used for donor egg treatments. These eggs may come either from another infertile patient; or a volunteer egg donor; or a friend or relative, who offers to donate eggs.

Egg donation for IVF or GIFT requires the egg donor to undergo ovulation induction and ovum aspiration. The donation of eggs carries more risk and causes greater inconvenience to the donor than does the donation of sperm.

The use of donor eggs requires that the cycles of the donor and the recipient be closely synchronized. Such synchronization requires treatment of the recipient, so that her endometrium is primed and is receptive to the embryos at the time of transfer. For women with ovarian failure, this can be achieved by treating them with exogenous estrogens and progesterone.

In the future, it is possible that scientists will discover ways to collect and store immature eggs. This may make "egg banks" a reality, and considerably simplify the technique of egg donation.

Risks and Complications of IVF and GIFT

The medical risks involved in any form of assisted reproductive technology depend on each specific step of the procedure. Ovulation induction carries with it a risk of the hyperstimulation syndrome, in which the ovaries become swollen and painful. Fluid may accumulate in the abdominal cavity and chest, and the patient may feel bloated and nauseated. About 10% of patients undergoing superovulation will suffer from a mild case of ovarian hyperstimulation syndrome. Of these, less than 1% would develop a case severe enough to require hospitalization. The condition tends to resolve itself unless pregnancy occurs, which may delay recovery. In IVF and GIFT, the hyperstimulation syndrome occurs less frequently. This is probably because the follicles are emptied of fluid and some cells during the egg harvest procedure.

Complications can also occur during the egg harvest procedure. Laparoscopy carries with it the risk of any surgery requiring anesthesia. The removal of eggs through an aspirating needle under ultrasound guidance entails a slight risk of bleeding, infection, and damage to the bowel, bladder, or a blood vessel.

In all techniques of assisted reproductive technology, the chance of multiple pregnancy is increased when more than one embryo or egg is transferred. Although some couples would consider having twins to be a happy result, there are many problems associated with multiple pregnancy, and these problems become progressively more severe and common with triplets and each additional fetus thereafter. Women carrying a multiple pregnancy may need to spend weeks or even months in bed or in the hospital. There may be enormous bills for the prolonged and intensive care for premature babies. There is also a greater risk of late miscarriages or premature delivery in the case of multiple pregnancies.

A recent treatment option for women with multiple pregnancies is that of selective fetal reduction, in which one or more of the fetuses is selectively destroyed (usually by injecting a toxic chemical, potassium chloride, into its heart under ultrasound guidance). In most cases, the killed fetus is then reabsorbed by the body, and the other fetuses continue to grow. Of course, the risk of all the fetuses being lost because of a miscarriage (as a result of inadvertent trauma during the procedure) is also present.

In addition, there is approximately a 5% chance of an ectopic pregnancy occurring with IVF and GIFT, the risk being more with GIFT.

IVF is physically demanding – and stressful! The effects of various blood tests, anesthetics and operations are tough on your body. Hormone stimulation causes lethargy and fatigue, notwithstanding the sometimes extensive travelling required each day. Some people find that the demands of IVF treatment conflict with the demands of their employment or other commitments.

A final risk involved in going in for IVF or GIFT is not physical, but psychological. Couples undergoing IVF and GIFT have described the experience as "an emotional roller-coaster". The treatments are lengthy, involved, and costly. These procedures often create high expectations but are more likely to fail than succeed in a given cycle. The unsuccessful couples will feel frustrated in their quest for pregnancy. It is common to feel angry, isolated, and resentful towards both the spouse and the medical team. At times, the frustration leads to depression and feelings of low self-esteem. The support of friends and family members is very important at this time.

Supporting Each Other

You may not be able to comfort each other enough at times of disappointment, especially when you are both upset. If you don't have a family or a friend who can provide support (without pressure), then the positive and sensitive assistance offered by a support group may be very suitable, either in the short term or long term. Other people may seek the more specialized assistance of a counsellor, who is either attached to the clinic or based in the community.

Selecting an IVF/GIFT Programme

When selecting an IVF/GIFT programme, information is crucial. Important points for consideration include the qualifications and experience of personnel, types of patients being treated, support services available, cost, convenience, and rate of successful pregnancies. Older programmes have established live birth rates based on years of experience. Although new programmes won't have as much experience and may still be determining their live birth rates, the personnel involved in them may be equally qualified.

Patient selection can influence the pregnancy rate. Some types of patients are more likely to become pregnant than others. For example, couples over the age of 40 and those with male factor infertility are less likely to get pregnant than are younger couples with tubal disease, minimal endometriosis, or unexplained infertility. The range of services offered by a programme should also be considered. Some programmes are equipped to handle sperm/egg donors and cryopreservation of embryos. Others may offer combined IVF-GIFT, ZIFT, PROST and TET.

The foregoing considerations and answers to the following questions, which may be asked of the programme, will help you make an informed decision when choosing an IVF/GIFT programme.

Cost and Convenience

1. How much does the entire procedure cost, including drugs per treatment cycle?
2. Do we pay in advance? How much?
3. What are the modes of payment?
4. How much do we pay if the treatment cycle is cancelled before egg recovery? Before embryo replacement?
5. What are the costs for embryo freezing, storage, and transfer?
6. How will the treatment schedule affect our commitments at work?

7. If we must have lodging, is there a low-cost place for us to stay? Do you help arrange this?
8. If I do not get pregnant, when do I make my next appointment for further evaluation and counselling?

Details about the Programme

1. How many doctors will be involved in our treatment?
2. To what degree can my own doctor participate in my treatment?
3. What types of counselling and support services are available?
4. Whom do I call day or night if I encounter a problem?
5. Do you freeze embryos (cryopreservation)?
6. Is donor sperm available in your programme? Donor eggs?
7. Do you have an age limit?

Success of the Programme

1. When did this programme perform its first IVF procedure? First GIFT procedure?
2. How many babies have been born from this programme's IVF efforts? GIFT efforts?
3. In the past two years, how many treatment cycles have been initiated for IVF? For GIFT?
4. How many deliveries resulted in twins or other multiple births?

24

Using Donor Sperm

THERAPEUTIC INSEMINATION BY DONOR (TID) means using the sperm from an anonymous donor to achieve a pregnancy. TID is a treatment option if the man is infertile – after all, when all is said and done, treatment for male infertility is still not too successful.

Getting Set for TID

Before a couple chooses TID as a treatment option, they must remember the taxing ethical, emotional and psychological repercussions it holds for both of them. The husband may feel threatened, isolated, inferior, insecure and jealous. He may wonder whether he will be able to play father to "another man's child".

The woman may be resentful that she has to undergo treatment and turmoil for something that is not actually her "fault". She may also worry about bearing the baby of a total stranger, and will often have no support, as this treatment may be something which is so private and secret, that she may not be able to share the truth with anyone -- even her own mother.

Couples undergoing TID are often subjected to psychological reactions which can be difficult to cope with. The sense of isolation is even more than with other forms of infertility, since most couples do not tell anyone they are undergoing TID. Consequently, they miss the social support and sympathy which other infertile patients receive. The stress can be tremendous because the sperm of another man are being inseminated into the wife, and both partners experience many conflicting emotions. The involvement of a completely unknown third party as a sperm donor can make coping with the pregnancy especially difficult. Fantasies and nightmares may occur about the unknown donor, and anxieties may arise as to whether the child would be normal and what the child would look like. Many men also experience sexual impotency at this time, but this is only a temporary phase.

Now is the time to talk and discuss matters frankly with each other, to achieve togetherness. Air out all your apprehensions with honesty and maturity. Discuss how you will make sure that you will both be equal partners in parenthood. The wife will have to reassure her husband with tact, gentleness and humour of her commitment to him. Love, patience and understanding are very important now – this is a time when the husband and wife need each other the most. Seek counselling from your gynecologist or fertility specialist. Discuss other choices too. Don't rush into "adopting" a sperm – explore the alternative options as well!

Who Are the Donors?

The donors are healthy men between the ages of 20 and 40, from a sound background, and usually graduates. Those who are healthy, with no family history of illness, are requested to provide a sperm sample for testing. This semen is analysed, and accepted only if it has superior qualities: preferably, a count over 100 million per ml; and motility of 70% to 80%. The donor's blood is checked to make sure it is negative for AIDS, hepatitis and STDs.

After liquefaction, the semen sample is mixed with an equal quantity of the cryoprotectant medium (a chemical

USING DONOR SPERM

which prevents the sperm from being damaged even at very low temperatures) and is loaded into plastic straws. These straws are uniquely coded and sealed and then placed in steel tubs of liquid nitrogen where they are frozen to -196°C. (Sperm can remain alive at this temperature in a state of suspended animation for many years – and perhaps, even indefinitely.) One day later, one straw is removed and thawed to see how the sperm have survived the cold (cryosurvival). Only samples which contain at least 20 million motile sperm are accepted.

The sperm are then kept in cold storage (sperm banking) in liquid nitrogen at -196°C for at least 3 months (the quarantine period), which is how long it takes for the HIV virus (which causes AIDS) to become detectable in a person's blood after infection. The donor's blood is then retested for HIV, hepatitis and STDs, and the infected samples are discarded. The others can then be used safely for TID.

Donors are paid a little more than conveyance costs – they are usually philanthropic men who have experienced fatherhood and want to make another couple happy. They are not allowed to produce more than 10 babies each and the doctors generally scatter the offspring so that the risk of half siblings unwittingly marrying each other is reduced.

Known Donors

Sometimes, couples wish to use a friend or a relative as a donor. However, there are many dangers in doing so. Over time, the donor's psychological make-up as well as the couple's relationship with him may change. This change could create social and legal problems in the future. Furthermore, the couple becomes dependent upon the donor's discretion to keep the insemination a secret. This is why using a known donor is not usually a good idea, however tempting the idea may seem initially.

Mixing Sperm

What about mixing the husband's sperm and donor sperm for artificial insemination? Many couples, with male factor infertility, wherein the husband has a low sperm count, will request that the donor and husband sperm be mixed together and used for artificial insemination. The reason they make this request is to make treatment by donor insemination more acceptable to them – so that they can feel that the child born could have been a result of the husband's sperm fertilizing the egg. However, mixing sperm is usually not a good idea. Not only does the sperm mixture have a lower fertility potential (because the infertile husband's sperm can reduce the quality of the fertile donor sperm), but it may also mean that the couple are not psychologically ready for the idea of donor insemination. In case a pregnancy results, this unpreparedness can lead to problems in the future.

The Treatment Process

Initially, the couple signs a consent form for TID after appropriate counselling. The doctor will need to ensure that at least one of the woman's fallopian tubes is open. To confirm this, the doctor may advise a hysterosalpingogram or laparoscopy.

The woman may be treated with fertility drugs to ensure ovulation. Daily vaginal ultrasound scans are done from day 11 of the cycle to view the evolution of the egg and discover exactly when the maturing follicle bursts.

For frozen sperm, a straw of the appropriate donor (who best matches the husband's physical traits) is picked out and rechecked under the microscope to ensure that the sperm are bustling with activity. The doctor matches the donor and the husband for height, build, hair colour, skin colour, eye colour, Rh factor and blood group.

Under sterile conditions, the donor sperm is injected through a plastic catheter into the cervix. The patient rests for about ten minutes and that's that. The husband is encouraged to be present at the time of the insemination— this is one way of ensuring that both the partners can be close during the process. Some clinics will even allow the husband to do the actual insemination himself, so that he feels more "involved". There is no reason not to make love shortly after TID if this is what the couple wants to do.

After each insemination a two-week waiting period has to be "endured" to find out if the procedure has been successful. The entire course is like an emotional merry-go-round — anticipation, insemination, menstruation, desperation, and then, hopefully, elation!

Success statistics tend to mimic nature. They are 10% in a 25-year-old woman in one cycle; so that over six treatment cycles, the chance of a pregnancy is about 60% in a 25-year-old, and only about 20% in a 38-year-old woman. It takes Nature time to make babies, and patience is needed. The chances of success are the highest if the female partner is young, has no fertility problem and the husband has no sperm. Irregular menstrual cycles or a history of endometriosis or tubal infection decreases the chances of pregnancy. Interestingly, pregnancy rates with TID are lower in women whose husbands have a low sperm count, as compared to those whose husbands have no sperm at all. The reason for this phenomenon is not entirely clear.

Once a pregnancy occurs, it is no different from any other normal pregnancy, and is exposed to the same risks of miscarriage and birth defects. If the patient changes her doctor, she does not even need to tell her new obstetrician that she has conceived by TID. He will never know, and the parents' names on the child's birth certificate will be the mother's and her husband's.

With TID strict confidentiality should be maintained, and the identities of the patients and donors should be kept secret. Historically, parents have kept TID a secret from the child and from friends and relatives. Unlike adoption, TID is not obvious to those who know the infertile couple. It is entirely up to the parents to tell the child the circumstances of his or her birth and most Indian doctors advise against revelation. However, there is always the burden of secrecy which the parents have to bear for the rest of their life.

Common Problems

- To tell or not to tell friends and family?
- The need to explain to employers and coworkers the necessity of repeatedly arriving late, leaving early, and taking time off, without being able to give a convincing reason.
- To deal with an erratic ovulation cycle caused by anxiety.
- To keep your sexual relationship on an even keel.
- To work out a plan when one partner wants TID and the other does not.

The Donor Semen Sample – Fresh or Frozen ?

Traditionally, gynecologists have used fresh semen samples (ejaculated recently) for TID. However, as summarized in the following box, using fresh semen samples for TID can be hazardous to the patient's health. It is best to use frozen, cryopreserved, tested samples from a sperm bank for TID. It used to be felt that pregnancy rates with frozen samples were poor as compared to fresh samples. However, recent studies have shown that if the frozen samples contain a sufficient number of motile sperm, pregnancy rates with fresh and frozen samples are comparable.

Disadvantages of Fresh Semen

- There are no records of the donors and no information as to their medical and family history.
- It is difficult to match the physical traits of the donor and the husband.
- Using known donors can lead to rocky legal, emotional and ego problems.
- The quality of the sample is always suspect, but beggars can't be choosers!
- It could be difficult to produce a suitable donor at the critical time and, occasionally, a treatment cycle has to run dry.
- The spectre of unwitting transmission of AIDS looms large since fresh semen cannot be tested for AIDS.

Advantages of Frozen Semen

- Only frozen semen samples should be used for TID, according to the American Fertility Society guidelines.
- No risk of transmission of STD and AIDS as the samples are quarantined for three months and the donors are retested.
- Around-the-clock availability; no scheduling bottlenecks.
- High quality product, since it is tested before and after freezing.
- Rh negative donors can be used for Rh negative women.
- Physical traits of husband and donor can be neatly matched.

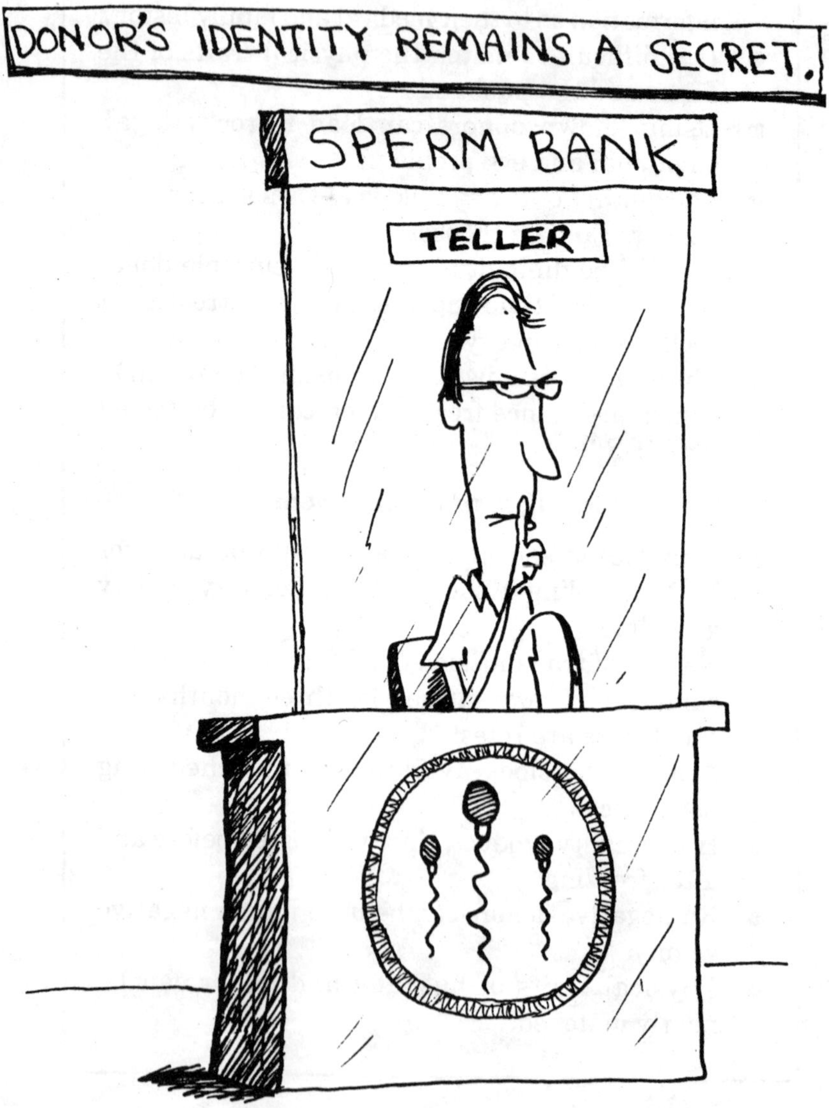
DONOR'S IDENTITY REMAINS A SECRET.
SPERM BANK
TELLER

25

Surrogate Mothering

THE WORD "SURROGATE" MEANS SUBSTITUTE or replacement and a surrogate mother is one who lends her uterus to another couple so that they can have a baby. In the West where fewer and fewer babies are offered for adoption, surrogacy is gaining popularity, despite controversial legal and ethical hassles.

Which kinds of women need surrogates? The commonest reason is a woman who has no uterus. The uterus may be absent from birth (Mullerian agenesis); or may have been removed surgically (hysterectomy for life-saving reasons, such as excessive bleeding during a caesarean section operation). Other women who may wish to explore surrogacy include those who have suffered multiple miscarriages, or who have failed to conceive despite repeated attempts at IVF for unexplained reasons.

Women who agree to become surrogates may do so for compassionate reasons. Such women could include a sister, mother or a close friend of the couple. They may also do so for financial renumeration, and this could be a woman, with or without children, known or unknown to the couple, who "rents" out her womb for a fee.

There are two main kinds of surrogacy:

1. The surrogate mother provides the egg. In this case, the surrogate is inseminated artificially by the

husband's sperm. Thus, the infertile woman has no genetic relationship to the baby.

2. More commonly, the infertile woman provides the eggs, which are then either transferred along with her husband's sperm to the surrogate mother's fallopian tubes by GIFT, or they are fertilized *in vitro* by IVF with her husband's sperm and the resulting embryos are then transferred to the surrogate's uterus, which then acts as an incubator for the next nine months.

Certain guidelines have been laid down in order to try to minimize misuse of the surrogacy technique and a surrogate motherhood contract needs to be drawn up, which should specify that the child will become the legitimate adopted child of the infertile couple, i.e., the intended parents. This contract needs to be signed by the couple, the surrogate, and her husband (if any), but cannot be held to be legally binding.

The "legal waters" of surrogate motherhood will continue to be murky, and, at present, no laws or guidelines exist in India. This is why the element of trust between the couple and the surrogate mother is so important.

It is vital that the surrogate and the couple consider the future of the child. The receiving mother should ideally be present at the birth and care for the baby in hospital. She can even be prepared for breast feeding by hormone treatment (induced lactation).

Surrogacy has spawned a host of legal and emotional questions to which there are no right answers. For example:

- What will you do if the surrogate insists on keeping the child?
- How much should you pay the surrogate?
- If the surrogate becomes seriously ill as a result of the pregnancy, who will pay the medical costs?

- Is it possible to put the receiving mother's name as the "mother" on the child's birth certificate?
- Will you tell the child about the surrogacy?
- Will surrogates undertake pregnancy merely for profit?
- What happens if the child is handicapped and is unwanted by the couple and the surrogate mother?
- What happens if the surrogate dies during child birth?

Many people are worried about the possibility of the surrogacy technique being misused. They feel it may allow the exploitation of poor women who may be used as "mother machines" to bear babies, much like the wet nurses of yesteryears.

Surrogacy has received quite a lot of adverse press publicity recently, especially when the contract goes sour and there is a dispute over the baby between the commissioning parents and the surrogate mother. Such a situation makes headline news. The courts then need to have the wisdom of Solomon to assign the rights of the "genetic" mother; the "birth" mother; and the "social or rearing" mother.

Nevertheless, we must remember that surrogacy does offer one method of achieving parenthood to a few couples who could never possibly have a baby by any other means.

The road to surrogacy is a rocky and uneven one and requires much thought and deliberation. This is perhaps the most complex and difficult way to achieve parenthood.

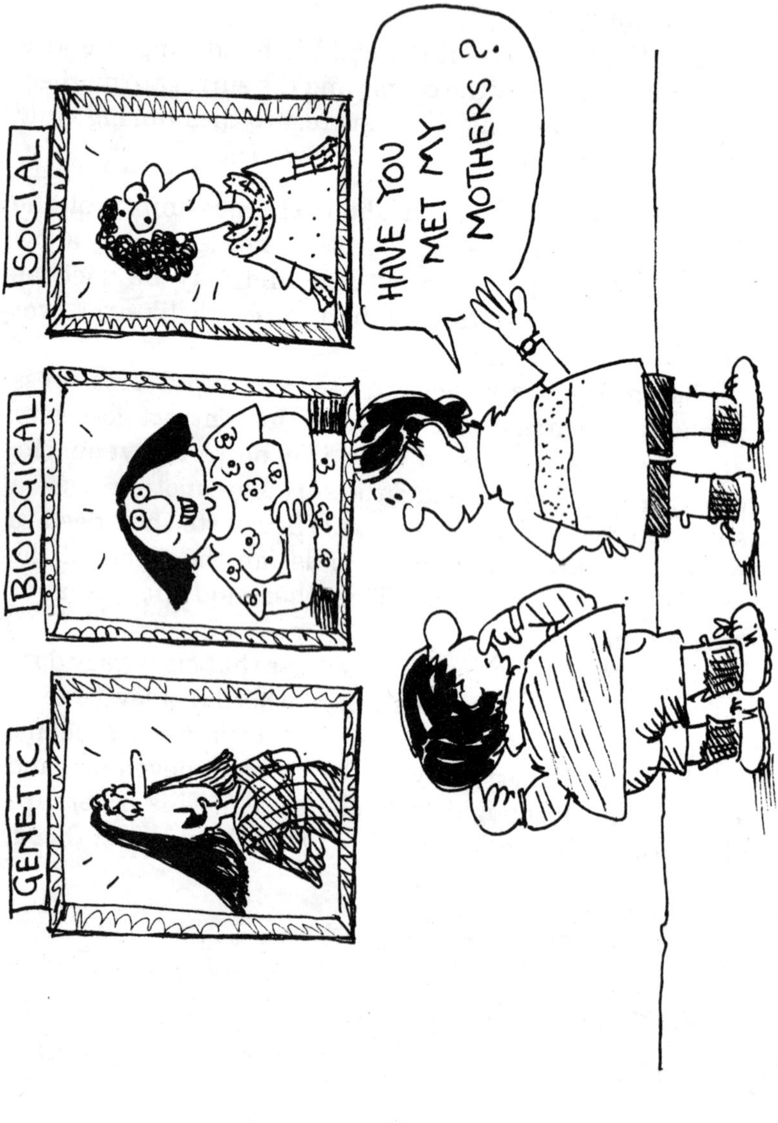
SOCIAL
BIOLOGICAL
GENETIC
HAVE YOU MET MY MOTHERS?

26

When Enough Is Enough – The Decision to End Treatment

ONE OF THE MOST DIFFICULT ASPECTS of infertility treatment may be examining the question of when to stop medical therapy. You may find yourselves asking: "When should we stop? When will we know that we have done all that we can?"

Only you both (as individuals) can tell when you have had enough – you need to make the final decision for yourself. Everybody has a different limit of endurance, but it needs courage to recognize when you have reached it. Some couples start planning for alternatives early on in medical treatment and when they feel that they have reached their limit, they are prepared to try something else. Others may keep going to a point which pushes them beyond their final limits – and sometimes even further!

Several reasons exist as to why infertile couples have trouble deciding when to stop treatment. First, there always seems to be a new medical option giving rise to fresh hope. How can you ignore a newly discovered course of treatment ("the latest advance") when you've been willing to try everything else? Some couples also seem to get "hooked" onto treatment, and are willing to give up everything to pursue their dream of having a baby – they live on hope. Another reason is that some physicians may not recommend ending treatment. Physicians are generally optimistic that treatment will eventually work and this factor tends to bias their ability to provide advice about ending treatment appropriately (to say nothing of their financial motives!). Some couples also feel guilty about stopping treatment even when they have had enough, because they feel they have let their doctor down by not getting pregnant – especially when the doctor has tried so hard!

How will you recognize the stage when you have had enough? Watch out for some of these factors:

- Do you feel emotionally weary and physically tired all the time?
- Do you feel sad or depressed much more than you used to?
- Are you finding it harder to be optimistic about your next treatment?
- Do you glumly anticipate a treatment's failure in order to fend off disappointment?
- Are you finding it harder to follow the doctor's instructions?
- Has your relationship with your spouse started to deteriorate even further? Are you fighting a lot more than before?
- Do you find yourself wondering why in the world you are doing all this?

There are positive reasons to consider ending treatment too – you don't have to wait till you are a wreck before making this decision !

- Are you beginning to focus more on the child, rather than on your genetic contribution to the child?
- Does the idea of stopping treatment seem to provide relief from your troubles?
- Are you directing attention to other areas of your life, and enjoying it?

- Do you feel proud of how hard you tried, and don't feel the need to do any more?
- Is your curiosity about alternatives increasing?

If you're considering ending treatment, you and your partner will probably find that one of you is ready to stop before the other reaches the final point. Remember, it's perfectly natural for people to move at different paces, especially through a process as complex and challenging as infertility and its treatment.

Facing the Final Decision

If you do find yourself faced with the decision to end fertility treatment, but you're not sure how to go about finalizing it, there are several steps that may help you determine what's best for you. Consider establishing a time frame. It sometimes helps to make a schedule for yourself, even if you decide to modify it later. You could decide, for example, that you will try for another year, or until your next birthday.

Another step that might be helpful is to take a brief "vacation" from treatment. Depending on your feelings after a break, you may realize that you're not ready to stop as yet; or that now is the time to end treatment.

Infertility, with its endless tests and treatments, has probably meant that so far your life has been put on "hold". But, through grieving and resolving your grief, you can move on again. Remember, you need to finish "mourning" for the loss of your child before making this decision. Grieving is letting go – letting go of unfulfilled dreams and replacing them with a comfortable reality, to allow resolution.

Talk to others who have decided to move on. An exchange of views is especially helpful if you are having difficulty deciding what to do next. Ask others how they made the decision and how they feel about it now.

Additionally, professional counselling can be very helpful in assisting you with decision making.

Finally, accept (and expect) that your infertility will remain a part of you. The decision to stop treatment brings resolution and closure, but it may not necessarily remove the ache and pain of infertility. However, once you do accept your decision, you may find that your disappointment gradually disappears.

WHEN ENOUGH IS ENOUGH

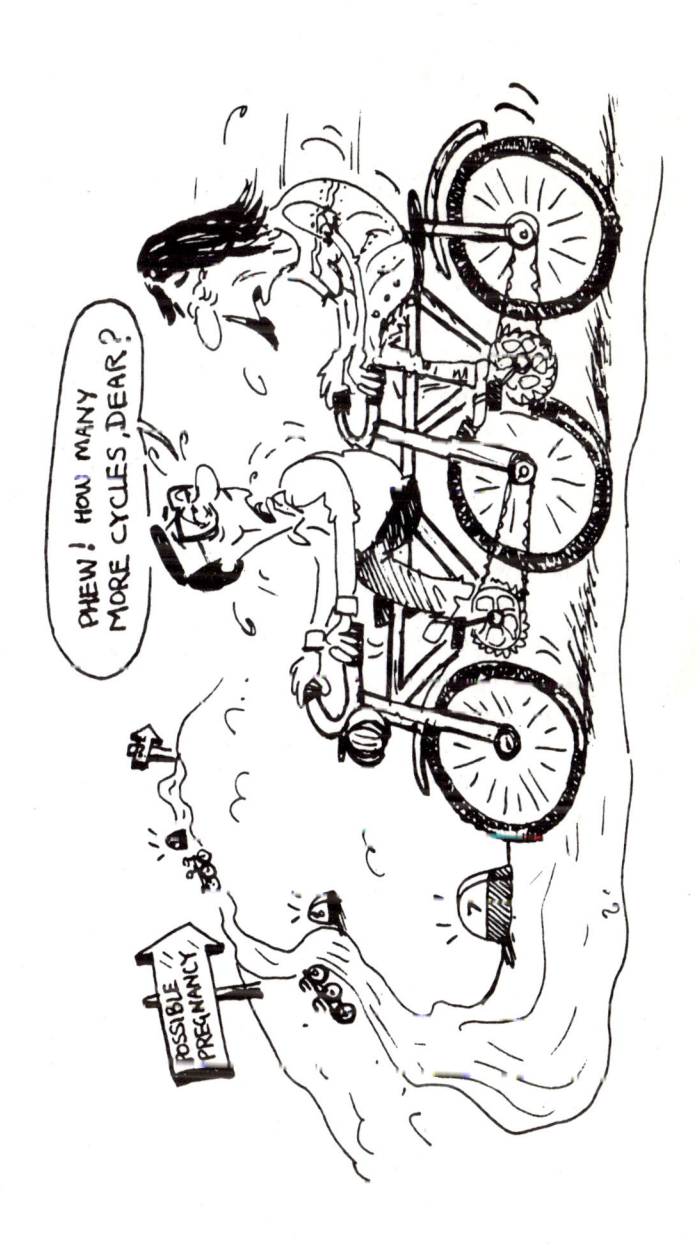

27

Adoption – Yours by Choice

YOU DON'T HAVE TO BE SUPERHUMAN, superkind, superloving or superperfect to be able to adopt a child – you just have to be ready. Being ready only happens when you've had time to get used to the idea; and if you are infertile, it is never too early to consider adoption. You can begin gathering information from adoption agencies even though you may not be fully committed. It is always a wise strategy to investigate alternatives in case pregnancy does not occur – after all, statistically, the overall chance of pregnancy for an infertile couple undergoing treatment is only about 50% to 70% after one or more years of trying. Also, because many agencies do not accept people over a certain age as adoptive candidates, especially for infants, it is important to collect information so that you don't discover later that you are too old to fulfil a particular agency's requirements.

To couples just beginning to consider adoption, the central concern is: can we love an adopted child as our own? Other doubts include:

- What kind of children are available for adoption? Aren't most of them misfits or discards?
- Won't adopted children grow up maladjusted?
- What will the reaction of our family members be? Will they love a child we adopt?

- Won't the child go off to find its birth ("real") parents once he or she grows up and discovers the truth?
- Why do we have to go through so much agony to build a family? Infertility was one struggle and now adoption with its waiting list is a whole new one.
- What will society think? Will our child be accepted by friends and neighbours?

As you find yourself more ready and receptive to accept adoption as an alternative, these questions often lose their importance. Some of them disappear when you finish grieving for your biological child — the child that never was — and overcome this grief by allowing the process of healing to occur. Through grief, you learn to focus less on the process of obtaining children and more on the children themselves. A couple must, together and separately, come to terms with their loss, to learn to say good-bye to their dreams of having a biological child, before they are ready to consider adoption. The other doubts disappear after you talk with adoption agencies; other adoptive parents and their families; read books about adoption; and learn how adoption is accomplished. The question then is no longer: "Can we do this?" but becomes: "How do we do this?"

You will learn that families with adopted children are the same as other families in many ways. You'll express love, have disputes and make compromises in your daily lives. Your child will be your child, no matter how you came to have him or her.

Adoptive parenting may be your second choice but it's just as good as biological parenting. The two experiences are, inevitably, totally different; don't try to compare them, one isn't better than the other. However, you will have to deal with several issues that occur only in adoptive families. Prepare yourself to discuss adoption with your child and to truthfully deal with the myths and misconceptions that many people have about adoption. You may also find that you and your child will often be faced with awkward questions and ignorant comments which assume that adoption is a second-best alternative for all involved.

Adoption cannot solve the problems associated with infertility; it is a cure neither for the physical aspects of infertility nor for the emotional pain. But adoption will provide you with the challenges and rewards of loving and being loved by a child.

Most adoptions are closed adoptions in which the biological parents and the adoptive parents do not come in contact with one another. The adoptive parents have only fragmentary, if any, information on the birth parents. Furthermore, adoption agencies make every effort to keep the adoption records confidential and unavailable to everyone, including the adoptive parents, the birth parents and the adopted child. Most agencies believe that the clear separation of the adoptive parents from the birth parents is necessary for the adoptive family to be "normal".

What is involved in the adoption process? Many people naïvely believe that adoption simply consists of walking into an agency and walking away with a baby. Of course, it's much more complex than that! Adoption involves considerable paperwork; asking questions; solving problems; researching; spending money; and going through emotional ups and downs. It takes time and work but remember that those who want to adopt will always succeed. The adoption procedures have been designed for your benefit; so don't be lured into taking "shortcuts" — these can hurt you in the long run. After all, adoption is not just a means of finding babies for infertile couples, but also a way of finding the right family for a particular child.

Each adoption agency has different requirements; so you may find that even though you are turned down at one agency, another one will readily accept your application.

ADOPTION – YOURS BY CHOICE

Most agencies suggest that:

- The age between the adoptive parents and the child be less than 40 years.
- The couple should have been married for at least five years to attest to the stability of the relationship.
- The couple should have a regular source of income.
- Neither of the partners should have a major illness which may reduce their life-span.

The professional who will be guiding you through the adoption process is normally a medical social worker, who is fully qualified and trained. Find an agency where you are comfortable with the social worker assigned to you.

You should learn about the requirements for adoption and also about the average waiting time for placement. You'll need to decide upon many factors including the child's age and sex – and there may be certain limitations on your choice. Costs vary widely, and you should enquire as to precisely how much expense you will have to incur.

Once an agency accepts your application, detailed interviews, both separately (with husband and wife), and jointly, are conducted. Agencies may ask you to supply references from relatives, employers and friends. Furthermore, an adoption worker will come to your house and evaluate your suitability as parents (called the home study). At some point after the home study period, a child is identified who is or who might be available for adoption. You'll then have to decide whether or not to accept the child – it's finally your choice. If you choose to adopt, there is a supervisory period once the child arrives in your home, and this may range from a few weeks to several years. After a specified period, your child can be legally adopted by you through an adoption decree from the court.

When Adoption Is Not the Answer

Infertile couples are often subjected to tremendous pressure to adopt. Friends and relatives may get tired of your infertility problem and question as to why you don't adopt if you want a child so badly. Others who have already adopted may enthusiastically recommend the option to you. But you should never try to force yourself to be comfortable with adoption if you find the idea to be disturbing – this is not a time for selflessness. There are no set guidelines to determine who should or should not adopt. Remember, adoption neither means trying to find a baby now to take care of you in your old age, nor is it a method to try to keep your marriage intact. Signs suggesting indecision could include denial of your disappointment about infertility; persistent fantasies about what life might have been with biological children; and the desire to keep the adoption a secret. Prospective parents may also have fears that an adoptive child may not measure up to family standards. If you have any doubts, it may be a good idea to temporarily postpone your adoption plans and discuss your anxieties with close friends or a counsellor before proceeding further.

Myths and Facts about Adoption

Myth: If an adoptive family really loves the child and does a good job of parenting, then an adopted child will not be curious about his or her birth parents.

Fact: Children are often curious about those who play major roles in their lives. Most, if not all, adoptive children will want to know about their biological roots.

Myth: Adopted children are better off not knowing they are adopted.

Fact: Adoptees almost always find out that they have been adopted. They then discover that their family has been dishonest with them. Adopted children may build better self-esteem when they have a clearer picture of personal birth origins.

Myth: Once the process of adoption is over, having an adopted child is the same as having a biological child.

Fact: There are real differences between birth and adoptive families. The adoptive child will have different questions about adoption at each stage of development.

Myth: Adoptive parents make better parents because they want a child so badly.

Fact: The intensity of desire for a child does not necessarily make for better parenting.

Myth: An adoptive child belongs to his new family forever and owes them something more than ordinary offspring.

Fact: An adoptee child offers neither more nor less to his parents than a birth child.

Myth: Once a couple has decided to adopt a child, it is more likely that the wife will then become pregnant on her own.

Fact: It is neither more nor less likely that a couple who has adopted will achieve a pregnancy.

Myth: Once adoption has taken place, the pain of infertility will cease.

Fact: The pain of infertility often lingers after the family has been established by adoption. Although happy with their adoptive families, couples may still want to pursue treatment for having a biological child of their own. Adoption is not a cure for infertility, but it can be a cure for childlessness.

Myth: Prospective parents should adopt only after all possibilities of having a biological child have been exhausted.

Fact: Because of rapid developments in infertility management, there is no longer a clear stopping point for possible infertility therapies. It is helpful for prospective parents to look into alternative means for starting a family early in their infertility work-up – remember, undergoing infertility treatment and considering adoption are not mutually exclusive choices! Just because you are undergoing treatment does not mean that you are not "committed to adoption"; and just because you are considering adoption does not mean that you are decreasing the chances of the infertility treatment as a result of your "negative attitude". Often, couples pursuing infertility treatment may actually begin to realize how an adopted child could be a good choice for them.

Myth: It is extremely difficult to adopt a child.

Fact: Although the adoption process can be tedious, adoption is possible for most couples.

Myth: Since India has an overpopulation problem, with so many unwanted children, adoption is a "better" choice for the infertile couple than taking treatment.

Fact: You cannot force someone to adopt a child, and adoption is not the best solution for all infertile couples. They need to be able to make their own choice. While adoption is a reasonable solution for some infertile couples, this is a choice which they have to make for themselves.

A useful book which provides more information about adoption is Nilima Mehta's *Ours By Choice*, which is available from the Family Service Center, Eucharistic Congress Bldg. III, 5 Convent Street, Bombay 400 039.

28

Child-free Living – Life without Children

CHOOSING NOT TO HAVE CHILDREN AT all is an option which you can select, i.e., to live child-free. Remember, child-free living is a choice you can make – choosing not to have children isn't the same as having childlessness thrust upon you.

You may find that coming to terms with your childlessness gives you the ability to take control of your own life again. Infertility often means living in a state of suspended animation – waiting seemingly forever through tests and treatments for a baby. If you choose to lead a child-free life, you can get on with living again. Plans can be made to explore the endless possibilities of career, travel, recreation, hobbies and togetherness as a couple when previously all the uncertainty engendered by the demands of treatment made this impossible. When you are chasing the dream of a baby, it is easy to forget that life has the potential for offering many other means of achieving satisfaction and fulfilment.

It is crucial, however, for both partners, should they choose the child-free alternative, to feel they can happily fill their lives with work and other interests. If the husband has a successful career but the wife has little to replace the parenting function, unhappy consequences are likely to result.

One of the biggest fears people express when considering a child-free life is that they will regret this decision in their older years and end up being lonely and miserable. In India, children are often considered a form of social security for old age. However, remember that children are not necessarily an insurance policy against loneliness in old age — they can also create problems for their parents! People also worry that when they die, they will have no progeny to leave behind to continue their lineage. The truth is that children are not the only ones who remember you, nor are they the only means of establishing everlasting memory.

Remember, there can be real advantages in leading a life without children: more personal freedom, more time to spend on your own interests, and more energy to invest in your emotional relationships. For example, you can start enjoying the time with your spouse more! Do you recollect the early heady days of your marriage before you were striving for a child? You can now try to recapture those magic moments again.

After opting for a child-free future, it may initially be difficult to adapt to a new life-style because of the multitude of new possibilities and choices now open to you, and many people advise that you try to do many things that interest you to give yourself a chance to expend some of your pent-up needs — the need to be needed and the need to do something worthwhile. It's a matter of balance, and you are free to choose. The answer to wanting one thing exclusively is to get involved in many things — to spread yourself around. Taking a holiday to mark the end of treatment and the beginning of a new life-style can be very helpful. Such a diversion provides time to relax in order to assess the situation objectively.

Acceptance or resolution of infertility doesn't mean regarding all desire to have children as bygone and forgetting about it. Your experiences and thoughts while dealing with the infertility problem will always be a part of you and will be remembered with mixed emotions over the years, including sadness, regret and frustration. Acceptance is more an acknowledgement that your hopes weren't to be realized and that you have to make some readjustments in life. This is not something you can do suddenly. You gradually come to this point, maybe over the course of your infertility tests and therapies, or maybe only when ultimately all courses of treatment have failed to produce any positive results.

The way in which different people cope with childlessness will depend on many factors, but the following should be borne in mind:

- There is no "right" way of coping with childlessness. Each person's way of coping will depend on his or her own experiences and emotions, and has to suit that individual.
- You have to give yourself time to get used to the reality of childlessness.
- There will be times when it will be more difficult to tackle life's problems than at others, and your level of coping will fluctuate. There are bound to be moments of doubt and questioning — what if ...?
- Denying that childlessness hurts doesn't help. The more you express your true feelings through tears, or by writing down your thoughts, or by talking, the easier it will become.
- You may feel angry because the thought of childlessness might be so hard to contemplate. This anger might be directed towards your partner, yourself, or your doctor. Recognize that such a situation represents a start towards acknowledging your feelings.
- Try not to apportion blame — there is really no one to blame.

- You should constantly remember that many others have survived this crisis and gone on to lead happy and contented lives – and so can you!

Even as you grow older, you may still find that other people treat you as "odd" or "different" because you have no children. You have to accept this situation and learn to live with the fact that you need not conform to others' norms in order to lead a happy life.

Creating a new identity without children is an important part of asserting control over your infertility. This process involves trying to think beyond children and deciding what you want for yourself. The only effective way to cope with childlessness is to build up your self-esteem which may have been battered by the agony and suffering experienced due to infertility. Creating a new identity does not mean abandoning your reasons for wanting a child. Just as those reasons shaped your infertility experience, so will they affect the form that your resolution takes. For example, you may choose to spend time with a children's organization as a volunteer.

Taking an interest in other people's children on a regular basis may also be helpful. When you were a child, remember how you longed to see that special auntie or uncle? Enjoy the company of children around you – use your energies constructively for a child that exists.

Another useful outlet for the longing to nurture children is to keep pets. Lovable and furry pets such as a dog or a cat are the most popular, because they can return your affection and love, but infertile couples have reported deriving pleasure from almost anything alive – from fish to flowers to gardens.

The passage of time serves as a healing process, but it can't be hurried. Time brings a sense of perspective or the "larger view of life" for those who have had tunnel vision focussed only on infertility for a number of years.

Soul searching can be helpful – and try answering the following questions together, honestly!

- Why do you want a child?
- Why would you not want to have a child?
- Think of the time before you tried for a baby. What made you happy? How did you spend your time? What did you look forward to?
- What are your other dreams and ambitions besides having a child?

Remember that the value of, and reward from, a firm resolution are what you make of it. If you select a child-free life, and then treat it as a second-rate existence, that's exactly what it will become. But if you invest it with all your interests, pleasures, energies and talents, this lifestyle can be creative fun, delightful and filled with accomplishment. Such a lifestyle may not be for everybody, but it may be just right for you!

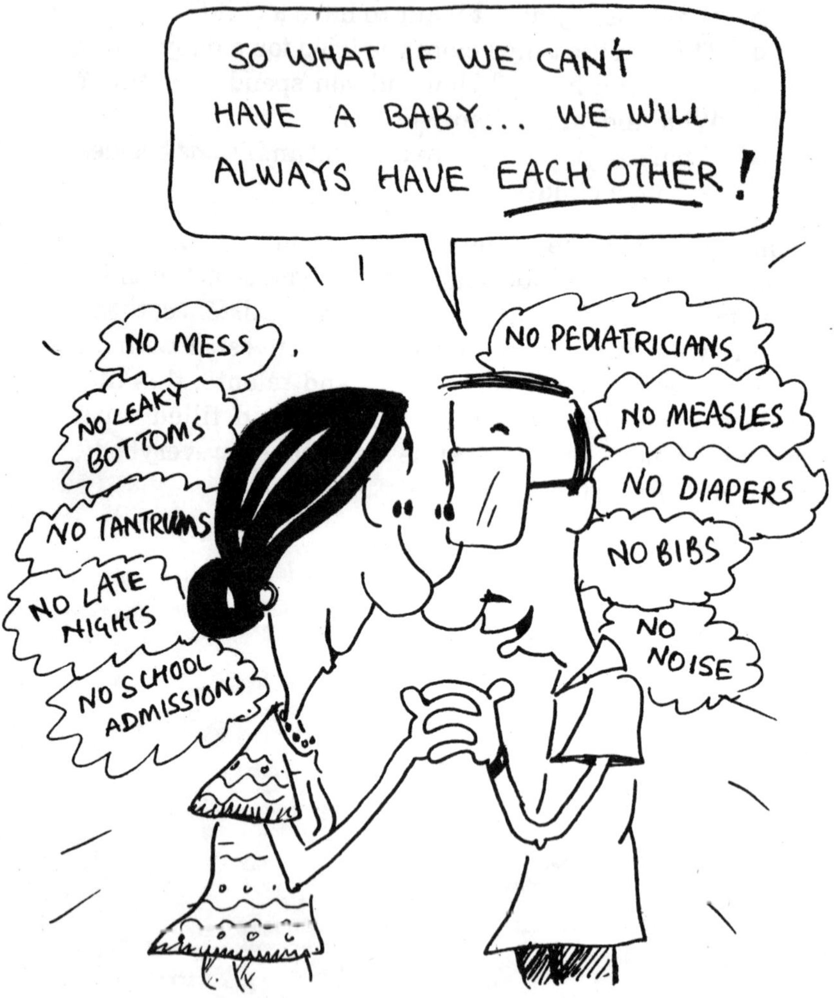
SO WHAT IF WE CAN'T HAVE A BABY... WE WILL ALWAYS HAVE EACH OTHER!
NO MESS
NO LEAKY BOTTOMS
NO TANTRUMS
NO LATE NIGHTS
NO SCHOOL ADMISSIONS
NO PEDIATRICIANS
NO MEASLES
NO DIAPERS
NO BIBS
NO NOISE

29

The Emotional Crisis of Infertility

SIR WILLIAM OSLER, A FAMOUS PHYSICIAN, once said that human beings have two basic desires – to get and to beget. To have your own family is a universal dream. This dream can become a nightmare for the infertile couple and learning that you have an infertility problem can engender painful and difficult emotions. Infertility is like a chronic illness that uses up a large amount of a couple's resources – emotional and financial – and involves the expenditure of a considerable amount of time, money, and physical and emotional energy.

Every person's response to infertility is different, depending on individual situations, emotional strengths, coping methods and personality. You will be confronted with the emotional impact of infertility before, during, and after treatment. It is better to prepare yourself for these difficult periods, so that with emotional support and mental preparation, you can successfully reduce the potential pain of infertility.

Discovering that You Have an Infertility Problem

Although you may have friends who have experienced infertility and you're aware that it is a common disorder, the news that you are affected by it is almost always unexpected. As you examine the issues surrounding

223

infertility, you may find yourself experiencing some uncomfortable emotions. Some of the most common ones are as follows :

Shock: In most cases, infertility is not diagnosed until after one year of unsuccessfully trying to conceive. Because of this time span, you may suspect that you have a problem before finding out for sure. For many couples, infertility is very difficult to accept. Most couples initially respond with feelings of shock and disbelief. After planning for years to have a child "one day", you may feel that your life's plan has been put on hold. These feelings generally only last for a short while and are not emotionally harmful if you recognize and deal with them.

Denial: Another part of the emotional process is often denial. You and your partner may find yourselves saying: "This can't be happening to us!" and, rather than confronting infertility, you may choose to deny the problem. However, this phase serves an important purpose and allows you to adjust to an overwhelming situation at your own pace as you work at resolving your infertility problem. Denial is only unhealthy if it lasts for a prolonged period and prevents you from accepting the reality of infertility.

Fantasizing: For some women, denial also leads to fantasizing — they dream of what life would be like if they had a child. They feel that all their problems would be solved if they got pregnant. They lose touch with reality and every time they start treatment, they think that they are going to conceive. They find it difficult to cope with the situation when the treatment fails.

Guilt: Guilt is an unfortunate, but common, response to infertility. In an attempt to determine why you are infertile, you may wonder if past behaviour caused the problem. Some individuals may feel that they are being punished for past sexual activities or an elective abortion. Often infertile partners may feel that they are depriving fertile partners of the opportunity of having children. The inability to produce a baby may also make you feel you have let your family down because you have not been able to fulfil what is expected of you, especially so if you (or your husband) are the only son or daughter of your parents. In large joint families, this stress can be stifling – and fertile daughters-in-law are given special privileges from which infertile women are excluded.

Bargaining: This is a common response, especially if you believe in god. You promise to fast; offer penance; offer money; and to be good for the rest of your life if god bestows the gift of a pregnancy upon you. Many infertile patients have visited an endless number of places of worship (such as temples, mosques) and "holy men", and have performed *yagnas* and *tapasya*, in order to conceive, often at considerable expense.

Blame: You may blame one another for your inability to conceive, especially when only one member is infertile. Also, you may respond differently to the emotional aspects of infertility. For example, one of you may find that the other is less concerned about having a child. As a result of these differences, one partner may grow resentful because the other is not experiencing the same emotions on an equal level.

Sadness and depression: The number of losses associated with infertility makes depression a very common response. In addition to the loss of a baby, infertility represents the loss of fulfilling a dream and the loss of a relationship that you might have had with a child. What you are mourning for is the absence of experience, and this type of sadness can be especially hard to deal with. You and your partner may have even more difficulty in dealing with these losses because friends and family often underestimate the emotional impact of infertility – and you have no one to talk to and share your burden with. The nature of infertility is such that you may never know definitely whether you are able to conceive or what precisely is causing the problem. Your grief, therefore, has nothing to focus on — and there is the continual hope that "this will be the time", which can leave your emotions painfully suspended, creating a continual "hoping against hope" attitude. When someone dies, the death brings family and friends together to grieve the loss, and this helps in healing. In contrast, infertility is a very private form of grief — you grieve alone without social support because the loss is hidden.

Hopelessness: Hopelessness is related to depression and usually results from the up-and-down cycle of emotions produced by infertility and its treatment. Most likely, you'll feel hopeful during midcycle when you've been treated and are looking forward to success. But if the cycle is unsuccessful, hopelessness can result, and you may feel that you'll never ever become pregnant. Starting all over again each month can make the process of dealing with infertility especially tough. After the disappointment of several unsuccessful cycles, you may find it difficult to maintain a positive attitude. You may think that it gets easier with the passage of time — but it never does. Every time that the treatment fails, old wounds (which you hoped had healed) open up again. After all, every time you start a treatment (especially when it is a new type of therapy that you have never tried before, or treatment by a new doctor), you always do it with the hope that *this time* it's going to work for you. If you didn't have this hope, no matter how small, you would never start treatment at all!

Loss of control: You and your partner have probably planned your lives so that you'll begin a family at the most favourable time. Many of us believe that everything is possible if we work hard enough — and not being able to have a baby is often the first time you experience failure against forces at work which are beyond your control, no matter how hard you try. You may have practised birth control for years and waited until both your careers were established before trying to have a baby. Discovering that you are infertile erodes these feelings of control over your own life. During treatment, you may find yourself putting other parts of your lives on hold. Such a predicament might include postponing moving to a new home, continuing your education, changing jobs, or establishing new relationships. The more you give up, the less in control you're likely to feel. Each treatment cycle can become a roller-coaster of emotions with its ups and downs — the hopes of success and the frustration of failure.

Anger: Anger arises from having to withstand a great deal of stress and bear many losses, including the loss of control. It is not unusual to be jealous of pregnant women, and to resent friends and family members who do not seem to understand the emotional tension associated with infertility. Often the anger is directed towards doctors, and this is one of the reasons why so many infertile patients change doctors so frequently.

Isolation: Feeling isolated is a common experience among infertile couples and coping with such isolation is even more difficult. Most people cannot comprehend the complex feelings associated with infertility. Insensitive remarks, such as: "relax and you'll get pregnant!", or "after you adopt you'll have a child of your own", are not based on fact and can cause a great deal of pain. It is not unusual for relationships to change if friends and family members are unable to understand, and empathize with, your feelings. Let your friends know that what you need is not their advice, but their support.

Infertility is an experience that continually fluctuates in intensity and direction, so that at different times you may feel different needs and experience different emotions. There are no set "stages" in this experience, and, while, at one time, your emotions can be mystifying and frighteningly intense, at another time, you may simply feel numb. There may be moments when the fact of being infertile dictates every facet of your life. The way you learn to deal with the experience of infertility will also be different at different times. One day a particular strategy may help you a lot, but later on you may find it useless. At times you may find that the pain you experience is very destructive, but at others you may find it a useful motivating force in your life. It is important to acknowledge that emotional responses to infertility vary greatly, as do different people's methods of coping with them. Each person has to find his or her own way of coping with the infertility situation, and sometimes might need help to accomplish this.

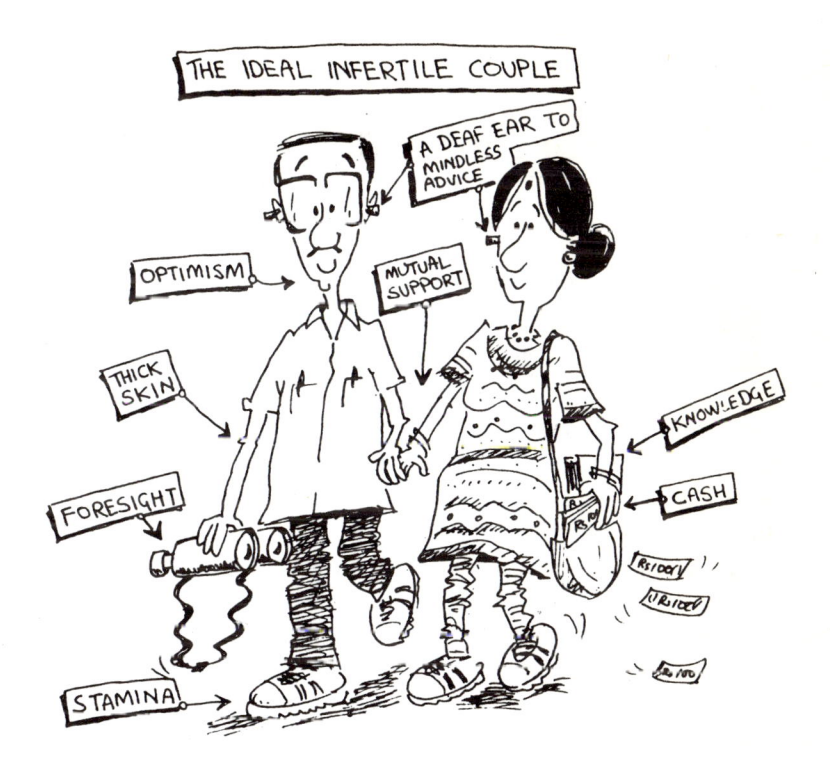

THE EMOTIONAL CRISIS OF INFERTILITY

30

How to Cope with Infertility

EVEN THOUGH THE STRESS OF INFERTILITY is often unavoidable, there are many steps that a couple can take to decrease the pain. First of all, both of you must recognize that you'll have different feelings and different reactions at different times. If you expect your partner to behave in a certain way, you may create additional stress. Together, you should become well informed about infertility and its treatment. Learn to focus on those factors which are within your control (for example, stopping smoking) rather than those over which you have no control (for example, your age). As you examine the treatment options and emotional stages, you can identify in advance the times when you will be facing difficult situations. Then, as a couple, you can plan to make such times easier. Discuss with each other your feelings concerning infertility and its treatment. Determine if your expectations of one another are realistic, and accept that differences of opinion may exist between you and your partner.

Sharing Your Feelings

Sharing your feelings with others is essential when dealing with the emotional aspects of infertility. At times, valued friendships are especially important, but friends and family may not understand what infertility means, and they will sometimes make insensitive remarks. As a result, feelings of isolation may increase, and this could lead to depression and loneliness. It is important to remember that others will never know what exactly you're going through unless you tell them. If friends make discouraging comments, try not to close them out. You may want to attempt to let them know how you feel and how they can help. Some of the following tips may be helpful:

- Don't assume that everyone understands your needs and knows precisely what you're thinking.
- Don't always put on a brave front. Friends and family may think that you are not distressed at all and don't need emotional support.
- Try to identify your feelings and share them. Putting your thoughts down on paper is often a helpful exercise.
- Offer friends and family reading material concerning infertility. Articles or books with quotes from individuals who have experienced the problems of infertility firsthand are especially beneficial.
- Become aware of your own anger directed towards your body, your partner, your relatives and your friends. It is important to recognize the effect of such anger on you and your ability to communicate with others.
- Examine your expectations of yourself and try to understand that infertility can lead to feelings of helplessness and loss of control.
- Examine your expectations of others. You will be disappointed if you expect others to always be there to support you.
- Accept your own feelings and acknowledge that there may be times when it is okay for you to avoid certain emotionally painful situations.

Coping with Infertility in Everyday Life

Undergoing treatment can "eat up" your entire day — waiting to talk to the doctor, waiting to take your injections, waiting for scans to be done, waiting for blood test reports and so on. The process seems endless and all you do is wait! The treatment seems to take all day — and you don't seem to have time to be able to do anything else. You need to take firm control of your time. While some waiting is unavoidable, a lot of it can be minimized. Can your husband learn to give you the injections so that you don't have to come into the clinic for them? Can you get the blood test reports on the phone? Learn to make good use of your time — you can keep yourself well informed about your treatment by reading about your infertility problem in books, magazines or journals while waiting. You may also find talking to other infertile patients about their experiences quite helpful, and the clinic often becomes the place for an informal "support group" meeting!

The waiting to get pregnant also makes you put the rest of your life on "hold" — you find you cannot make plans for the future because you do not know what lies ahead. Should you plan to go on a holiday next month — what if you get pregnant? Should your husband accept the new job, even if it means a transfer to another city where you will have to find a new doctor? Such dilemmas can be frustrating — not only are you not getting pregnant, but also you cannot get on with the rest of your life! You need to try to separate infertility from other important aspects of your life, and remember that you are otherwise a worthy person, irrespective of your fertility. Women often have a harder time coping with infertility, because they have been taught that their life revolves around their family, which has yet to be started! Often, getting a job is helpful, because it keeps you occupied and bolsters your self-esteem by confirming what you know — that you can accomplish useful feats in your life, irrespective of your infertility.

Talking to relatives and friends can be difficult when they ask awkward and thoughtless questions about infertility. Some typically painful questions and comments include:

- So when are you going to start a family? You two aren't getting any younger!
- When are you going to stop concentrating on your career and start on a family?
- Well, I guess we'll never be grandparents.
- Oh, I have just the opposite problem – I get pregnant so easily!
- I wish you'd take one of my kids – they drive me crazy!
- I hear they're having tremendous success with test tube babies. Why don't you try it?
- You can always adopt.
- Any good news yet?

Questions and comments from others can sometimes be turned into opportunities for you to explain your situation more fully to them; or else you can discourage further discussion. Be firm and pleasant, and don't let yourself be put on the defensive. After all, just because a question is asked does not mean it deserves an answer, so with a smile, you can let the others know that it's none of their business without being rude yourself.

Think about how you will respond to these questions, and plan ways in which you can successfully manage the conversation. There are emotional barriers between the fertile world at large and infertile couples – and you need to work to overcome these barriers!

Times that May Be Especially Difficult

Social gatherings such as weddings, where the conversation generally focusses on pregnancy and children, can be difficult to cope with. You'll also inevitably have some friends who become pregnant during your infertility treatment. The news that infertile friends have conceived with treatment can be bitter-sweet – you are happy for them, and know that this also means there is hope for you. Nevertheless, you feel it's unfair that you are not the one who got pregnant, and sometimes despair whether you will ever be able to have a baby. Furthermore, certain holidays, birthdays and anniversaries may generate added stress by reminding you that time is passing by without your having children.

Time becomes the enemy – whether it is the incessant ticking of the biological clock, or the apparently endless waiting for the next menstrual period. The few days before your next period is due can be hell for both of you. The suspense can be killing – and you await every day with bated breath to see if the period has started. Each twinge of pain or drop of discharge is monitored carefully – and if the period is delayed, hopes of pregnancy start rising. Then, when the menstrual flow starts, all the castles built in the air come crashing down, and you become inconsolable. You sometimes start wondering whether it is worth beginning all over again?

Coping with treatment is difficult too, especially when you know that it is impossible to predict the outcome for most treatments. Also, with Nature's imperfection and today's technology, the chance of your not getting pregnant in any one cycle will always be more than the chance of your conceiving. Often, the key to success may be to repeat the treatment several times but this can be pure torture! You need to be realistic about your chances of conceiving – this level-headedness can act as a buffer to minimize the disappointments and tribulations of failure. Some women feel that they must maintain a "positive" attitude, no matter what, and put up a brave front to the world. But merely pretending to be hopeful when you are broken inside increases your burden.

Regaining Control

In order to decrease your feelings of helplessness and to regain control of your emotions, there are several things you can do. First of all, devote time to learning about your infertility. By doing this, you will feel more in control at your doctor's office and you'll be better able to understand the tests and procedures that you're undergoing. Read about infertility treatment, and discuss your ideas and opinions with your physician. It's also important to talk with all your health care providers. For example, the nurses attending to you may be able to help you with troublesome emotions as well as medical questions, or a technician could explain test procedures and results.

You need to make an "action plan" outlining possible courses of action as regards your medical treatment. For each treatment cycle, hope for the best and prepare for the worst. If you get pregnant, that's fine; but you should know what do next if you do not, so that you are not shattered when the treatment doesn't work. Many couples refuse to think about the possibility of failure and plan treatment on an *ad-hoc* single cycle basis. This is unrealistic and you are only fooling yourself. Being realistic allows you to cope with the ups and downs of treatment, and you need to have a perspective which spans four to six treatment cycles, so as to give yourself a reasonable chance of success.

During treatment, you need to set your own limits. Sometimes, treatment becomes a merry go-round, which never appears to stop and you find that you just can't get off. Some patients get "hooked" onto treatment and never give up, at great pain, agony and expense to themselves. Decide when you will stop treatment and which treatments you will try. This is a decision only you can make and you should be satisfied that you have done all that you want to, so that you do not have any residual feelings of regret or recrimination later! If medical therapy becomes too stressful, consider taking a break. When necessary, make it a point to remind friends and family that these are your decisions and that you *do* know what's best for you.

Little things that you can do for yourself can make a big difference in how you handle your infertility. Write down positive things you have done or good things that have happened to you, and read this list often. Plan a special evening, and share your thoughts and feelings with your partner. You and your partner may want to join a support group so that you can meet people who are experiencing similar infertility problems. It is also important to become more informed about infertility, so that you can share this information with friends and family members who do not seem to understand the stress and pressure accompanying this disorder.

Many patients find religious support at this time is very helpful; and a deep belief and abiding faith in god can help you immensely in tiding over this crisis in your life. Others use meditation to help themselves.

How Infertility Affects Couples

Infertility is a medical problem that involves two people, and both of you remain involved even if only one person needs medical treatment. Attend medical appointments together if possible – it can be very lonely and frightening sitting alone in the doctor's office, and the support you give to your partner by your presence is very helpful. Sometimes, the partner who is undergoing all the tests and treatment (usually the woman!) may feel resentful and angry at all the poking and prodding done to her body. Blow your top – but not at your partner – rage at fate instead. Chances are that your spouse would do anything to take over this burden from you. If you are the partner who is not being treated, you may feel strangely guilty that you are getting off "free". You may also be upset and blame your partner for the infertility problem; but being upset and apportioning needless blame are two different things. Some husbands are very upset about all the procedures that their wives have to undergo, and often cannot bear to see the pain they have to suffer.

Men and women generally respond differently to infertility. Generally, while men are definitely concerned about infertility, it may be less crucial to their self-esteem and identity. Also, handling the emotional impact of infertility may be more difficult for men because they are not used to voicing and sharing such types of concerns and anxieties. They are taught to bottle up their feelings. On the other hand, women frequently accept the label of being infertile as a key aspect of themselves and who they are. In Indian society, the pressure to conceive is directed towards the woman, and it is often she who has to bear the brunt of its impact.

It is common among infertile couples for the woman to be the much more emotional and verbal partner. This often leads to the wife thinking and talking incessantly about infertility, and her whole world now revolves around how to have a baby. She talks (or sometimes complains or screams or cries) about it and wishes her husband could feel the intensity of her pain. He tries to be supportive, but never seems to be able to do or say the right thing; so he gets put off and shut off and refuses to talk about the problem, thereby exacerbating the tension even more. In order to help keep infertility from becoming an all-consuming catastrophe and to break this vicious cycle of one-sided conversation in which no productive communication occurs, the "20-minute rule" recommended by Merle Bombardieri of the USA, an infertility counsellor, is very useful. You need to set aside a period of time each evening to talk about infertility. Use a timer to limit each person to 20 minutes and let one speak and then the other. The person not speaking needs to listen intently.

The foregoing technique is useful in achieving the following outcomes:

1. The wife will talk less about infertility and will present her feelings more succinctly.
2. The husband is more willing to listen because he is assured of an end point.
3. The wife feels she has an interested listener and is being supported.
4. The rest of the evening may be spent in more pleasant pursuits.
5. You may both feel relieved to see the other feeling better.
6. In all likelihood, as the wife feels she has less need to talk about infertility, the husband will begin to be more expressive, so that the wife no longer needs to "grieve for two".

Communication in your relationship may change as you and your partner deal with infertility and its treatment. Sometimes, you may keep your emotions to yourselves as you try to protect one another from painful outbursts. This situation may create especially difficult feelings such as anger, blame, and guilt, and you may find that there is even more pressure on your relationship. You have the right to feel differently about infertility treatments and choices – after all, even though you are a couple, you are still individuals with your own separate identities. Individual responses depend upon individual personalities, coping mechanisms, who has the fertility problem, and your relationship with your partner. You may feel hopeful and optimistic, while your partner feels hopeless and despondent, and you may find that you are balancing on opposite sides of an emotional seesaw. You can agree to disagree, but keep your heads cool, and if you fight, fight fairly and honestly without hurting one another.

You may discover that learning to cope with infertility allows you and your partner to grow and mature emotionally and come closer as you share your feelings throughout this difficult time. As an additional bonus, your marriage becomes stronger than most marriages because you have weathered a difficult time together successfully.

When Professional Help May Become Necessary

If you remain constantly depressed, rather than experiencing periods of "ups and downs" that seem to be related to your treatment, you may need to seek professional therapy. Counselling can help you to honestly and sincerely examine your feelings, determine your priorities, and improve your coping skills.

There are several signs that indicate serious depression. If you find yourself constantly feeling sad, desperate, worthless, or inadequate, professional counselling may help you better understand your situation. Other signs that indicate a need for professional counselling are lack of motivation, withdrawal from social activities, feeling overly sensitive, vulnerable, or guilty, and having suicidal thoughts.

In addition to the emotional signs of depression, there are several biological and physical signs that you should look for. For example, if you're having difficulty falling asleep or staying asleep or if you find yourself waking up early and being unable to go back to sleep, this could signal depression. Other signs are excessive increase in, or loss of, appetite, loss of sexual desire, and undue fatigue.

You might also want to seek help if you and your partner are unable to communicate with each other about the infertility problem and its treatment, and if you're having difficulty coping with extreme anger or resentment.

It is important to select a therapist who has adequate experience in infertility treatment, and can effectively help you in dealing with the difficulties and emotions that go along with it. Remember, you have to choose the therapist. It is acceptable to interview a number of professionals in order to select someone who is familiar with your situation and who makes you feel comfortable.

Your physician may be able to recommend a suitable therapist, or you may want to check with a professional medical or psychological organization, or an infertility support group in your community, in order to seek appropriate counselling.

31

Infertility and Sexuality

INFERTILITY BRINGS ABOUT MANY CHANGES in a couple's relationship. It may bond you both closer together in unspoken sadness and hope, and may also engender mutual support and understanding which lead to a sharing of emotions never before experienced. On the other hand, infertility may bring out feelings of resentment, of guilt, and of despair. As the initial months of investigations turn into frustrating years, it is not surprising that sex quickly loses many of its associations with fun and pleasure and instead becomes a chore with a single-minded purpose.

Failure to conceive certainly destroys self-esteem, self-worth and sexuality. All the negative feelings are reflected in the bedroom, which is, after all, where all the "problems" started.

The psychological effect of a diagnosis of infertility on sexuality has largely to do with one's self-image. Fertility is one very basic expression of sexuality. Even today, the man with six sons, in many countries and cultures, occupies a higher status than a man who has borne none, because he is considered to be more potent and more virile.

The emotional response to a diagnosis of infertility is a "grief reaction". Infertility involves many losses: those of potential children and the family planned and dreamed about; genetic continuity; the experience of conception, pregnancy and birth; the gift of grandchildren to one's own parents; the central meaning of one's life plan and marriage; and the procreative potential in sexual relations. It is common for a woman to feel "less of a woman" and a man to feel "less of a man", at least for some time, when faced with the reality of infertility. Many men describe feeling like a "dud" or "sexual failure" (and may use other expressions relating to feeling emasculated).

Women, too, often feel their sexuality threatened when faced with the possibility of not becoming pregnant. Women are probably more powerfully socialized than men into the expectation that they shall conceive and become mothers in the normal course of events. When this process is thwarted, there is often the feeling of having failed as a "proper woman", as revealed in the following statement (of a woman who had undergone several treatments for infertility):

> I saw the blood (of the menstrual period) today. I feel weak and tearful. All the strength I'd thought I'd acquired just seems to have drained away. The discomfort serves as a reminder of my failure. For many women menstruation is a sign of femininity and potential for motherhood. All it signifies to me is my failure.

Here is a comment about sexual attractiveness:

> I have always been told I was pretty. I liked the way I look, and I felt confident in social situations. After my pelvic surgery, the doctor told me he had never seen a worse mess of adhesions in his life. He said it looked like a little kid had been let loose with a pot of glue and stuck everything all together. I am ugly on the inside and pretty on the outside. I would gladly have the reverse if it would make me have a baby.

There are four significant periods which impinge on the feelings about sexuality for the couple faced with infertility. These are:

1. When trying to get pregnant.
2. During investigation and diagnosis.
3. During treatment.
4. Menopause.

Let us consider each period separately.

When Trying to Get Pregnant

The usual advice given to a couple trying to start a family is to have unprotected sexual intercourse for at least twelve months before having fertility investigations. This waiting period can be nerve-wracking! Doubts about one's fertility almost always result in a heightened awareness of signs of fertility that surround us. Pregnant friends, noisy children in markets, media coverage of new reproductive technologies, hints from eager parents wanting grandchildren — all these factors can begin to erode the sexual self-confidence of the couple wishing to have children. Inevitably, sexual intercourse is timed during the fertile time of the woman's cycle. Spontaneity goes out of the window as the sexual life of a couple comes to be associated month after month with the aim of procreating and the failure to conceive. Men often come to feel like a "stud bull", and women may feel it is pointless to engage in sexual activity when it is unlikely to result in pregnancy.

During Investigation and Diagnosis

Those not faced with infertility would be staggered by the number, complexity, and invasiveness of medical procedures that a couple with a fertility problem go through in their search for an answer as to why pregnancy is not occurring. As one patient put it: "It's like donating your body to science while you're still alive!"

A basic procedure is the basal body temperature chart. Although useful from a medical point of view, this chart also means surrendering some very personal information about oneself, as shown by this quote:

There is no inner recess of me left unexplored, unprobed, unmolested. It occurs to me when I have sex, what used to be beautiful and very private is now degraded and very public. I bring my chart to the doctor like a child bringing a report card. Tell me, did I pass? Did I ovulate? Did I have sex at all the right times as you instructed me?

The temperature chart begins to rule and ruin a couple's sex life. It is also a public declaration of making love. With the desire for a child becoming increasingly frustrated, life can become an endless maze of temperature changes, ovulation calculations, timing of sex and eventually the disappointing signs of one's menstrual onset. Anxiety, depression and fighting over sex can often be traced to this source.

As one "victim" of the BBT chart stated: "Ordinarily my husband was the instigator of sex. During my fertile time, I felt I had to seduce him. What quite often happened was that we'd end up fighting instead of making love."

And the husband felt: "It was pretty hard to feel an urge to make love when your wife is expecting a command performance."

It is not just the physical charting but the mental charting (which may continue indefinitely) that is a source of stress, even if the patient is not aware of what precisely is happening.

Some of the comments about temperature charting are quite telling:

> One of the things that made me freak out about charting my temperature was the accompanying need for the X's. I guess that is what brought home to me the fact that we had stopped making love as frequently as we used to.
> The ultimate moment for me was when I found myself cheating on the charts. I put in a few more X's here

and there to make things look good...then I said to myself: Good heavens – has it come to this?
At first it was quite exciting – I felt as if I was actually doing something. We would both look at the chart and go for, say, six X's in a row – in fact, our frequency of intercourse increased I'm sure. By now we've gone through the stage of saving up sperm and have hit the stage of almost total abstinence. I put in an occasional X so that the doctor or nurse doesn't get the impression that there's something wrong with our marriage.

Providing a sample for semen analysis can also be stressful for the husband:

I looked around desperately for something to turn me on – there was nothing – not even soap. After 15 minutes I gave up – literally sore as hell.

Most men feel their masculinity is "on the line" when having a semen analysis done, sometimes to the extent of being unable to produce the required specimen. It is not uncommon for the man to become impotent for a short time while he is undergoing such procedures : "The first time it happened I thought – here it is – middle age. I'll never get it up again."

While postcoital tests are painless and physically unobtrusive, many couples find them very difficult to undergo because they intrude so much on their intimate relationships. There's the need to comply with a specific time, the rush to the clinic to keep the appointment, the embarrassment and real fear of "failure" if all does not proceed as had been "instructed":

They told us to make love first thing in the morning and then come to the clinic. Well, what if you don't feel like it? We're dreadful in the morning. We put the alarm on at 6 o'clock and we had the kettle on to make coffee... making love was the last thing we felt like doing... he hated it and I hated making him do it.

The power play dynamics in the doctor-patient relationship takes on a new dimension when fertility is being investigated. Couples are desperate to find an answer to their difficulties and hence are compliant and rarely let the clinician know they are under stress ("not coping"). They must expose the most intimate aspects of their lives – their sexual relationship in their desire to have children:

> There's a coyness about the way doctors handle sex. It's as if infertility has nothing to do with sex, yet it has everything to do with it. I never know whether I want them to assume that I don't have problems, or whether I want them to ask me if I do have any difficulties.

During Treatment

A couple's decision to commence an infertility treatment programme, such as IVF or donor insemination, signifies their hope and excitement that they can overcome infertility, and produce children like everyone else. However, like the investigative period, this again signals a further, if not more intense, invasion of their sexuality and sexual relationship.

With each IVF cycle, women are confronted with multiple barriers to becoming pregnant, to becoming mothers, and thereby expressing a major aspect of their "femaleness". The low pregnancy rate – about 15% per treatment cycle – means that most women will leave the programme with a reconfirmed sense of failure, at least for a short time, and certainly if they have received little emotional support.

The use of donor sperm to start a pregnancy, as in a donor insemination programme (when the male partner is infertile), brings home to the man his inability to reproduce. Some of the feelings of inadequacy may have been worked through during the period following diagnosis, but it is not uncommon for these feelings to be rearoused when the programme actually begins. At most infertility clinics, the men are encouraged to be present while their wives are being inseminated. Some men even perform the insemination themselves (a painless and simple medical procedure). This encourages bonding between the couple at this crucial time, and especially gives value to the participation of the husband in the act of the conception of their child.

With respect to nearly all forms of infertility treatment, rarely is the infertility cured, and clearly not in cases where donor egg or donor sperm is used. For example, women with blocked fallopian tubes, who become pregnant after an IVF cycle, still face further IVF attempts if they wish to become pregnant again. A feeling of defectiveness may remain despite pregnancy and a live birth.

Menopause

Menopause is a time when all women are confronted by their sexual identity, simply because the physical signs of being a woman are changing forever. It is a difficult time of adjustment for many women, and for those affected by infertility, it means saying goodbye, yet again, to motherhood.

It is useful to ventilate feelings of frustration, anger and the feeling of being "taken over", as your sexuality gets trampled upon throughout the course of investigation and treatment. This will restore a sense of personal worth. Remember that it is normal, expected and almost inevitable that your sex life will take a beating for some time.

It is useful to join a support group or to talk to a counsellor who can help you to separate sex from reproduction. You can do this for yourself, too, perhaps by throwing away the temperature chart for a while, or by taking a break in the middle of a treatment programme to enjoy a romantic holiday.

32

Support Groups – Self-Help Is the Best Help

INFERTILITY CAUSES GREAT PERSONAL SUFFERING and distress. Most of the agony and misery is hidden from the public gaze, and that is why this topic is still not talked about openly. The reasons for the lack of public support for the infertile couple include the dismal ignorance about the causes of infertility and its treatment; and the failure of infertile couples to make their problems (and the solutions to them) known to the public, because of their low self-esteem and reluctance to talk about their experiences, thus leading to a vicious cycle.

Infertile couples are socially isolated and emotionally very vulnerable. They need a place or forum where they can get together and talk to people in the same predicament as themselves, so as to help them tide over this crisis in their life. After all, if infertile patients will not look after their own interests, then who will?

An organization called Infertility Friends is India's first support group for infertile couples. This is a non-profit registered charitable trust for infertile couples, where they can get together and discuss their problems. In order to facilitate this process, the patient education library contains over 30 videos, 50 books and 100 brochures, pertaining to infertility, which help patients in learning more about their problems.

The mission of Infertility Friends is to provide compassionate and informed help to people experiencing the crisis of infertility, and to increase awareness about infertility issues through public education. Its goals include: providing in-depth, reliable medical information which would encourage infertile couples to make informed decisions regarding the different treatment options available to them; encouraging patient self-education, resulting in a stronger doctor-patient relationship; and offering emotional support services to reduce anxiety and help restore feelings of self-worth, optimism and control over one's life.

How does a support group help? No one understands infertility as well as someone who has already been affected by it. However, finding another couple experiencing the same problem as yours can be difficult. Infertile people simply have no way of finding one another, and this is where support groups can provide help. Contact with other infertile couples is one of the best ways to break through the barriers of isolation and despair created by the infertility experience. You realize that "you are not alone" in your misery. By joining a support group, you learn that there are others who can understand the devastation of a failed cycle or the jealousy generated by a friend's pregnancy. The craziness of scheduled sex, the exhaustion of endless medical treatments and the agony of family gatherings are all well known in a support group.

The best help, of course, is self-help; and an additional bonus many people find is that by helping other infertile couples in their time of need, they learn to help themselves! Being able to ventilate your feelings and to get emotional support can prove to be a healing experience.

Unfortunately, misconceptions about support groups prevent many people from making use of this valuable source of help.

Some couples are concerned that joining a support group might cause them to dwell even more on their infertility. But the reality is that infertility can pervade every aspect of your life; and an obsession with getting pregnant will grip you whether you join a group or not. Trying to shut out painful feelings will only make them worse.

Others may feel that infertility is too private or personal or traumatic to share with a group of strangers. You may also believe that you should be able to handle this problem on your own. In truth, infertility is too traumatic not to share with others, and there is nothing wrong or weak about reaching out for help. A support group simply provides a safe, warm, supportive environment – you need never say a word if you don't want to.

Another reason for not joining a support group is the lurking fear that it promotes a feeling of futility. The perception may be that a group is only for those who have hit rock-bottom or are without hope. This is far from the truth, and, in fact, many support group members have ended up with successful pregnancies – thanks to the information that they obtained from the support group's library.

It's easy to believe that nothing except a successful pregnancy will make any difference in coping with infertility, but, again, that's also not true. Joining a support group may be just what you need to find crucial information or to deal with the devastating feelings that accompany being infertile. Joining may be frightening – but it's well worth the risk. You do not have to struggle alone.

The address of Infertility Friends is:

Infertility Friends
Jamuna Sagar
Bhagat Singh Road
Colaba
Bombay 400 005.

Additional useful sources of information abroad include:

Resolve, Inc.
1310 Broadway
Somerville, MA 02144-1731, USA.

The American Fertility Society
2140, 11th Avenue South
Suite 200
Birmingham, AL 35205-2800, USA.

Ferre Institute Inc.
258 Genesee Street
Suite 302
Utica, NY 13502, USA.

Infertility Federation of Australasia
PO Box 426
Erindale Centre
Wanniassa ACT 2903, Australia.

Child
PO Box 154
Hounslow, TW5 OEZ, UK.

ISSUE
509 Aldridge Road
Great Barr
Birmingham B44 8NA, UK.

The Endometriosis Association
8585 N 76th Place
Milwaukee, WI 53223, USA.

33

Myths and Misconceptions about Infertility

M *yth*: Painful periods cause infertility.
Fact: Painful periods do not affect fertility. In fact, for most patients, regular painful periods usually signal ovulatory cycles. However, progressively worsening pain during periods (especially when this is accompanied by pain during sex) may mean you have endometriosis, which may cause infertility in some women.

Myth: Infrequent periods cause infertility.

Fact: As long as the periods are regular, this means ovulation is occurring. Some normal women have menstrual cycle lengths of as long as 40 days. Of course, since they have fewer cycles every year, the number of times they become "fertile" in a year is decreased. Also, such women need to monitor their fertile period more closely, since this is delayed (as compared to women with a 30-day cycle).

Myth: Blood group "incompatibility" between husband and wife can cause infertility.

Fact: There is no relation between blood groups and fertility.

Myth: "The reason I'm not getting pregnant is because most of the sperm leaks out of the vagina after intercourse."

Fact: Loss of seminal fluid after intercourse is perfectly normal, and most women notice some discharge immediately after sex. Many infertile couples imagine that this overflow is the cause of their problem. If your husband had his climax inside you, then you can be sure that no matter how much fluid you lose afterwards, enough sperm will reach the cervical mucus. This leakage is *not* a cause of infertility.

Myth: You'll get pregnant if you keep on working at it and want it badly enough.

Fact: Unlike many other parts of your lives, infertility may be beyond your control. While newer methods of treatment have improved most couples' chances of having a baby, some problems still remain unsolvable.

Myth: Just pray and have faith in god.

Fact: Believing in god can help you in maintaining a positive outlook; but sheer will and blind faith won't overcome a physical problem like blocked tubes or absent sperm.

Myth: A man can judge his fertility by the thickness and the volume of his semen.

Fact: Semen consists mainly of seminal fluid, secreted by the seminal vesicles and the prostate. The volume and consistency of the semen are not related to its fertility potential, which depends upon the sperm count. This count can be assessed only by microscopic examination.

Myth: Infertility is hereditary.

Fact: If your mother, grandmother or sister has experienced difficulty in becoming pregnant, this does not necessarily mean you will face the same problem! Most infertility problems are not hereditary.

Myth: A retroverted ("tipped") uterus causes infertility because the semen cannot swim into the cervix.

Fact: About one in five women will have a retroverted uterus. If the uterus is freely mobile, this is normal, and is not a cause of infertility. Such a condition is *not* an indication for surgery!

Myth: We should be having intercourse every day to achieve pregnancy.

Fact: Sperm remain alive and active in cervical mucus for 48-72 hours following sexual intercourse; therefore, it isn't necessary to plan your love-making on a rigid schedule. Although having sexual intercourse near the time of ovulation is important, no single day is critical. So, don't be concerned if intercourse is not possible or practical on the day of ovulation.

Myth: A woman ovulates from the left ovary during one month and the right ovary during the next month.

Fact: Ovulation occurs from only one ovary during each month. However, the pattern may not be regular from side to side.

Myth: Pillows placed under the hips during and after intercourse enhance fertility.

Fact: Sperm shall already be swimming in the cervical mucus as sexual intercourse is completed and will continue to travel up the cervix to the fallopian tube for the next 48 to 72 hours. The position of the hips really doesn't matter.

Myth: If you just relax, you'll get pregnant.

Fact: If pregnancy has not occurred even after a year of trying, chances are that a medical condition is causing infertility. There is no evidence that stress causes infertility. Remember, all infertile patients are under stress; it's not the stress which causes infertility, it's the infertility which causes the stress!

Myth: Periods that occur at less than or greater than 28-day intervals should be considered irregular.

Fact: The length of each woman's menstrual cycle differs, and can vary from 3 weeks to 6 weeks. As long as a woman can count on a period at a regular interval, this is considered normal.

Myth: "I've never had symptoms of a pelvic infection, so I can't have blocked tubes."

Fact: Many pelvic infections do not cause any symptoms at all, but can nevertheless cause severe damage, which is sometimes irreversible, to the fallopian tubes.

Myth: "My gynecologist has carried out an internal examination and said that I am normal; therefore, I should have no problem getting pregnant."

Fact: A routine gynecological examination does not provide information about possible problems which can cause infertility.

Myth: If a woman takes fertility drugs, she'll have a multiple birth.

Fact: Although fertility drugs do increase the chance of having a multiple pregnancy (because they stimulate the ovaries to produce several eggs), the majority of women taking them have singleton births.

Myth: A man's sperm count will be the same each time the semen is examined.

Fact: A man's sperm count will vary as a result of several factors, and many of these are still poorly understood. For example, sperm number and motility can be affected by time between ejaculations, illness, and medications.

Myth: "I have no problems in having sexual intercourse. Since I am virile, my sperm count must be normal."

Fact: There is no correlation between male fertility and virility. Men with totally normal sex drives may possess no sperm at all.

Myth: All doctors are equally interested in the treatment of infertility.

Fact: Not all doctors or even all infertility centres share similar interests. It is important for you to ask your gynecologist about the treatment choices he can offer you and what the pregnancy results are following such treatment in his practice.

Myth: Infertility treatment should not be offered in India, because there are already too many babies in this country. Why increase the population problem by producing more?

Fact: The right to have children is a fundamental right of every human being and a very basic biological urge. Just because a neighbour has too many children, this situation should not deprive the infertile couple of their right to have their own kids.

Myth: Azoospermia (having no sperm) is a result of excessive masturbation in childhood.

Fact: Masturbation is a normal activity which most boys and men indulge in. It does not affect the sperm count. You cannot "run out" of sperm, because these are constantly being produced in the testes.

Myth: If the couple is infertile, it is a result of their "misdeeds" – infertility is the consequence of the couple's faults.

Fact: Infertility carries a major social stigma and therefore "victim-blaming" is very common, partly because most people know so little about their own fertility. However, a person's fertility is not really his or her control. You are not to blame if you have a fertility problem – it's not in your hands!

Myth: Infertility is not a medical illness and treatment should not be covered by insurance.

Fact: Infertility is a medical problem, which is often amenable to medical treatment. Insurance should cover the treatment costs.

Myth: IVF and related advances in infertility treatment are too expensive for Indians to afford.

Fact: IVF and related technologies are undoubtedly expensive; but then, so is heart surgery! Yet, no one objects when over Rs 1 lakh is spent to try to salvage the heart of a 70-year-old man (whose life expectancy in any case is only about five years and is not extended by the surgery). Why then should medical technology not be used to help couples in their thirties (with their whole lives ahead of them) have their own baby? In fact, IVF is a much more cost-effective use of medical resources than a number of other accepted surgical procedures (such as joint replacement surgery or kidney transplants).

Helping Hands – How Friends and Relatives Can Help

THE OBJECTIVE OF THIS CHAPTER IS to help friends and family members to understand better the problems and uncertainties faced by an infertile couple. Sometimes it's difficult to know what to say to a couple who are confronted by an infertility problem because it's such a private matter, that you'd rather not intrude. And, sometimes, it seems as if no matter what you do or say, it's the wrong thing.

Here are a few suggestions which may help you to provide the support and understanding that an infertile couple need:

1. Be ready to listen. Infertile couples have a lot on their mind and need someone sympathetic to talk to – to help them get things off their chest.
2. Don't offer advice unless you are very well informed on the subject. You may not be sure what their specific medical problem is, and, in any case, if they need medical advice, they can get it from their doctor.
3. Be sensitive and don't joke about infertility. Remember, infertile couples are hypersensitive about many things – try to put yourself in their shoes.

4. Be patient. Infertile couples are involuntarily caught in an emotional roller-coaster and often their moods and actions are unpredictable. Don't get hurt when they seem to be preoccupied with their own problems and are not paying adequate attention to you; they are not rejecting you — they just want to be left alone.
5. Be realistic and supportive of an infertile couple's decisions. Once they've reached a difficult decision, support them, no matter what your personal feelings may be. After all, this is their decision, so don't say things like: "I'd never consider doing that!"
6. Don't criticize their doctor or treatment choices. This only serves to aggravate their stress.
7. Understand that individuals and couples respond to infertility differently. Accept them for what they are, as they are, and where they are.
8. Above all, be there when they need you and show them that you care.

Remember that there is rarely a quick or simple answer to infertility problems. Assessment and treatment procedures usually take considerable time. You can help by not forcing the issue with questions such as: "How soon are you going to have a baby?" The couple may not know if they can have a child, much less when it will be born. You can help by allowing them to decide if and when they want to talk about it.

Each individual couple's experience of infertility is very real for them and cannot be compared with others as being more or less serious. The wish to have a baby, and the fear that it might not be possible, take on paramount importance. You can help by not comparing them with other people you may know about. Refrain from telling stories about other infertile couples — they are rarely helpful.

It is neither helpful nor medically sound to offer advice such as "relax" or "take a holiday". You can help by not giving misguided, albeit well-intended, advice. By being well informed, you can also help in breaking down the myths that surround infertility problems.

Some people consider infertility to be an extremely private concern. Yet others find comfort in being able to share their experiences with close friends and family members. It is normal for infertile couples to feel sad, angry or depressed at times. You can help by respecting their need for privacy, or, by offering support if there is a need to talk about it. Be prepared to accept the expression of feelings such as anger, sadness and depression.

Those experiencing infertility often feel inadequate because they have no control over their reproductive system. You can provide support by recognizing this fact and helping them to perceive their strengths, qualities and achievements in other areas of their lives.

Some people experience infertility problems after having one child (secondary infertility). This situation proves devastating and frustrating for those who feel their families are incomplete. You can offer support by understanding what this means to them. Avoid thoughtless comments such as: "You're lucky to have at least one child!"

Your encouragement, understanding and support for your infertile friends or relatives can help to guide them on their long road to resolving their infertility. This support could prove crucial to their emotional healing.

35

Making Decisions about Treatment

DISCOVERING THAT YOU HAVE A FERTILITY problem can be a difficult process. In addition to the emotional stress, you both now find yourselves faced with making endless decisions about treatment. (The word "decide" comes from a Latin root meaning "to cut away from".) Thus decision making, by its very nature, involves loss, giving up one or more options, while grasping others. Not deciding maintains the illusion that you can have it both ways – that there is no loss, no risk. Unfortunately, most infertile couples have not learnt to make their own decisions, and not making decisions is, in one sense, the worst possible decision of all! You cannot allow your doctor to make treatment decisions for you either – this can be disastrous as well.

Identifying Your Goals

It is most likely that your original goal would have been to have your own biological child. However, because of your fertility problem, you may be forced to examine your deepest feelings about family, children, and parenting. You could find that you have to re-evaluate your initial plans in order to get the family that you want.

As you work to identify your goals and examine your options, you'll discover that, essentially, there are four

MAKING DECISIONS ABOUT TREATMENT

choices as regards treatment. Depending on the cause and treatability of your infertility, you may need to choose one of the following options:

- To pursue the course for having a biological child through medical evaluation and treatment.
- To try to have a child biologically related to only one parent, either through donor insemination or egg donation.
- To adopt a biologically unrelated child.
- To decide to remain childless.

You may want to rate each of the four options as "desirable", "acceptable", or "unacceptable" at the beginning of your evaluation and periodically re-evaluate these choices.

For some infertile couples, trying to have a biological child and childlessness (child-free living) are the only options. For others, the switch from having a biologically related child to adopting or having a child biologically related to only one parent may be easier than having no children at all.

Many couples lose track of the fact that their main goal is to be parents, even if they can't be biological parents. Therefore, they may pursue infertility treatment for several years and find themselves above the age limit to adopt an infant through an agency. Furthermore, since a woman's fertility decreases after the age of 35, this also decreases the chances of successful treatment. You and your physician should try to take these possible consequences into account when evaluating and choosing your options.

If you are young (the wife is less than 30 years of age), there may be a good chance that you will achieve pregnancy without going in for expensive treatment procedures, such as IVF and GIFT. Therefore, you may not wish to explore these possibilities as yet. However, if you are older (the wife is more than 35 years old), you have less chances of conceiving, and a more aggressive treatment approach might be called for, since time is at a premium.

The decision-making process is different for each couple and depends on individual situations and personalities. For example, some couples may opt for expensive, high-tech treatments, while others in the same situation will wait to see if they can become pregnant without treatment.

What Kinds of Treatment Are Available?

Once you've discussed your infertility problems with your physician, you'll find that there are a number of treatments available, which include the following:

- Medication, which may be prescribed for either partner to improve fertility.
- Surgery, to correct an anatomic impediment which impairs fertility.
- *In vitro* fertilization (IVF) or gamete intrafallopian transfer (GIFT), for patients who require assisted reproductive technologies.
- Donor insemination, if male infertility is the problem.
- Egg donation, if the female cannot produce eggs.
- Surrogate parenting, if the woman has no uterus.

Questions You Should Ask Your Doctor

Your doctor may be able to make several useful recommendations about treatment, but there are a number of questions that you should always ask your physician so that ultimately *you* can make the best decision for yourself. Unlike other medical questions, infertility recommendations are not always clear. You need to evaluate whether or not each treatment option will help you reach your goals, and how well it will do so. After that, you'll have to determine which options you will pursue. The following

MAKING DECISIONS ABOUT TREATMENT

questions may help you build up a foundation of medical information to assist you in your decision-making process:

- How much will this treatment improve our chances of achieving pregnancy?
- How much risk is involved and what kind of risk is it?
- How long will we have to undergo this treatment in order to give it a reasonable chance to work?
- Will undertaking this treatment eliminate other options?
- How much will the entire treatment cost?
- Are there other options available if this treatment fails?

Your physician can help you determine how much time, physical discomfort, and risk would be involved and how much money will need to be invested in a particular treatment option. You will then have to decide how much money you are willing to spend, and how much emotional stress you can withstand.

You need to design your own fertility treatment plan. Not only will this plan help you maintain control over your life as you proceed with treatment, but it will also help in ensuring that you get good quality medical care — after all, a lot is at stake!

Issues Affecting Your Choice of Treatment

Issues which can affect your choice of treatment include the following:

Medical factors:
- Diagnosis (or lack of one).
- Quality and availability of medical care.
- Success rate of treatment.
- Level of technology required.

Personal factors:
- Age.
- Time commitment needed for treatment.
- Personal feelings (physical and emotional).
- Partner's feelings.
- Job and career.
- Financial resources.
- Ethical and religious concerns.
- Reactions of family members and friends.
- Other obligations and commitments.
- Willingness to change life-style.
- Aggressive or low-key approach to resolution.

Remember that there are no right or wrong decisions about resolving your infertility. Counselling may be helpful in setting out your priorities, especially if you and your partner disagree on the course of action. As your options change with time, you may also change your priorities. Try to be as realistic and open-minded as possible.

In order to make the impact of infertility treatments less stressful, you'll need to place time limits on them. Such a step may help you to define your goals more clearly. Many couples are willing to accept only two to three years of therapy, because continuing treatment for long periods of time may cause excessive stress.

It is important that you do not lose sight of, or in any way jeopardize, your relationship with your spouse. Make sure that each of you understands how the other feels about each stage of treatment. Throughout treatment, both of you may encounter times of ambivalence about having children. This is a normal reaction, and you should remember to have realistic expectations from one another.

If reasonable goals are maintained and each other's difficulties, anxieties and limitations are kept in mind, stress can be minimized. If this is not the case, then a break from treatment, a change in plans, or counselling for stress and marital issues may be a good idea.

Sometimes, recording information on a worksheet can be helpful. You may want to take each of the options your doctor has suggested, gather the relevant information that you need, and go over the options in terms of the following factors:

- Time.
- Physical risks and emotional stress.
- Cost.
- Chances of success, with and without treatment.

Also keep in mind how much money and time are needed, what financial resources are available and how much you are willing to invest. As you go through this decision-making process, you will probably find that your answers change with time.

If you do not conceive after pursuing your initial plan of treatment for a set period of time, you may need to re-evaluate your goals and options. You may find that you want to discontinue medical intervention, or you may want to seek a different kind of treatment. Keep in mind that it is not at all unusual for partners to have differing views and feelings about infertility and its treatment. Open communication can help both of you to make the best decision.

Facing Treatment

An early step in the entire process is to try and prepare yourself for the trials and tribulations ahead. Ask yourself if it is worth the risk of pursuing treatment without a guarantee of success. Anticipating difficult situations and emotions may help you deal with them more easily.

Your doctor can provide you with relevant information on treatment options and can refer you to further sources (such as specialists in the field of infertility treatment). You can take steps to prepare yourself for what could be a long and frustrating process. But you may also find that as you and your partner work through the stages of infertility treatment, your relationship tends to grow stronger.

Your physician, support groups, other couples who have made similar decisions, and counsellors can also provide support and guidance. Above all, remember that with patience, a positive attitude, and the appropriate treatment, most infertile couples *can* eventually become parents.

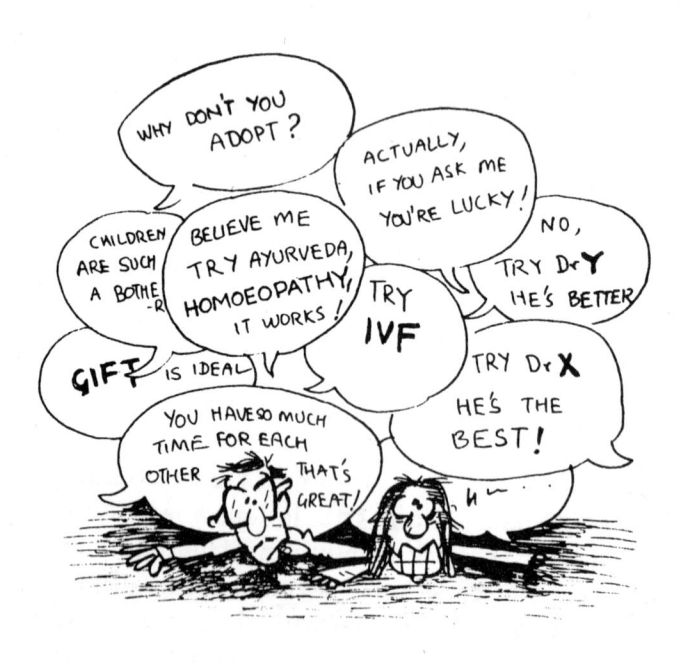

36

Your Role on the Medical Team

IN A PERFECT WORLD YOU WOULD have the perfect infertility specialist who treats you as an intelligent couple, who has plenty of time, infinite wisdom, low fees, no other patients, is totally honest yet compassionate, has a conveniently located clinic and understands your emotional as well as medical problems.

Since it's unlikely that you are going to find such a doctor, you have to do your homework to find a second best choice!

You can find a suitable doctor through:

- Professional referral. Ask any reliable doctor you know for suggestions.
- Friends, other infertile patients, and infertility support groups. These can also be helpful sources of information.

Selecting a Suitable Doctor

Selecting a suitable doctor can be difficult! Try to find answers to the following questions about any doctor you wish to take treatment from:

- What are his credentials (training and qualifications)?

- What about his skill and experience?
- Is he accessible (locations; clinic timings)?
- Is he affordable (fees)?
- Is his approach professional? Does he:
  prepare in advance for your appointment?
  discuss records and explain test results?
  keep appointments and value your time?
  manage an efficient clinic?
  review your status and progress periodically?
- What about his personality and style? Does he:
  talk patiently to you?
  take time to listen to what you have to say?
  show empathy and compassion?

A good infertility specialist will usually:

- Involve both husband and wife in consultations, discussions and planning.
- Offer worthwhile recommendations and choices. Since there are no "right" answers, he should allow you to choose your own course of action.
- Tailor testing and treatment to your emotional needs and budget.
- Devote time to answering questions and offering support, whenever needed.
- Chalk out a treatment plan for you, with a discussion of rationale, alternatives, costs, time limits and expected success rates.

Ultimately, you have to trust your doctor's skills to provide you with the best treatment for your infertility – that is why selecting the right doctor is such a crucial decision!

Most gynecologists can provide basic infertility workup and testing – but you may prefer to look for a specialized infertility clinic which will provide all the services that you need under one roof, especially if you have a complex problem.

Getting a Second Opinion

Get a second opinion – this can never hurt and is always helpful. If you find two experts holding the same view, then you know that you are on the right track! If, on the other hand, they disagree with each other, don't get upset because there are very few black-and-white areas in infertility, and different doctors often have different ways of treating a particular problem. Ask questions of both of them and then choose the method which appeals to you – it's finally your decision!

What if you don't understand what the doctor is trying to explain and are getting confused? This is not your fault. If you do not understand anything that the doctor says, do ask questions! If you still do not understand the fault is the doctor's; he is not explaining in terms which you can follow. You may be better off looking for another doctor!

Remember that you need to ask questions to get answers – your doctor cannot read your mind! But also remember that your doctor does not have all the answers – after all, medicine is still an imperfect science, and your doctor is not a fortune-teller! If the doctor does not know the answer, he should tell you this as well.

As an infertile patient, you are very liable to exploitation, and quacks in this field abound! Start suspecting your doctor's credentials when:

1. He promises too much.
2. He says things like: "That's my secret."
3. He doesn't explain clearly what he is doing during treatment.
4. He advises too many tests and surgical procedures repeatedly.

When to Change Doctors

Because infertility is often a long drawn-out process, anger is a natural result, and often this anger is directed towards your doctor. However, constantly changing doctors or "doctor-shopping" can be counterproductive! If the quality of care you are receiving is good, be cautious about changing doctors – a doctor who knows you and your infertility problems well can be of significant help to you. However, you should consider changing doctors if you are experiencing the following:

- Treatment without diagnosis.
- Lack of progress over time.
- Apparent lack of a treatment plan or disagreement about the treatment plan.
- Minimal communication from your doctor.
- Minimal attention to your needs and concerns from your doctor.
- Loss of confidence in the doctor's skill and knowledge.

The Need for Active Participation

Remember, you are in charge of your own medical care! Medicine, as both a science and an art, often requires choices, and there are really no "right" answers. Consequently, you need to make your own decisions. After all, it's your body and your life!

You have a vital interest in treatment decisions and outcomes but lack the medical knowledge and skill to decide alone. The concept of a team – the medical caregivers (doctors, nurses, specialists) and you (the couple) working together – allows each to contribute to a successful outcome and offers you a sense of control over your infertility care.

Your role on the medical team is multifaceted – you need to wear many hats when you are an infertile patient!

Medical information researcher: The more knowledgeable you are about your problem and its treatment, the better are your chances of getting pregnant. Educate yourself – you need to become an informed participant in your infertility care in order to ask the right questions and to get involved in making decisions about your treatment. You will also need to be able to critically assess press and media reports about "new breakthroughs in infertility treatment" and whether these new developments are relevant to your problem or not. An infertility support group reference library can be very helpful. A friend who is a doctor can also help in separating the wheat from the chaff.

Medical team manager: Remember – you are the one in charge! You will have to locate, choose, evaluate and sometimes "fire" members of the medical team.

Treatment decision maker: Although your doctor may be better equipped technically to select treatments, the ultimate decision rests with you. Each new treatment phase requires new decisions – you need to allow yourself time to choose from the different options available and to be comfortable with your choice, before starting a new treatment.

Treatment monitor: You are the "expert" on deciding what is normal for you – so, record and report reactions. Combining medical and patient information helps in improving the odds for successful treatment.

Medical record keeper: You must keep a record of all your tests, operative notes, reports and documents. Such a record can be very helpful if you need to change doctors or get a second opinion. File all records in reverse chronological order and also prepare a one-page summary sheet of what you've been through.

Financial manager: Infertility treatment can be very expensive, and, sometimes, it seems to be an endless drain on your financial resources. You must be aware of the costs involved, and you need to decide if you can afford these expenses.

Communicator: Because infertility involves extremely personal matters such as reproduction and sexuality, people sometimes find it embarrassing to discuss their concerns and worries. It is important that you be open and honest with your doctor. Ask questions, listen to the answers and take notes. It often helps to write down your questions before your appointment, so that you do not forget crucial doubts and concerns during the stress of the consultation. Remember, the only stupid question is the one you don't ask – so don't hesitate to ask !

Your Rights

1. You have the right to be treated in a humane manner with care, consideration and dignity.
2. You should be given a clear and concise explanation, in non-medical terms, of your problem by your doctor.
3. You should also be given a clear and concise explanation of the treatment or investigation conducted, including whether such treatment is of an experimental nature; or is empirical (of unproven value, based on practical experience).
4. You have the right to have your partner with you in the consulting room.
5. You are entitled to refuse an examination, a particular treatment, or an operation.
6. You have the right to ask for a second opinion. Ask the specialist you are consulting, or your general practitioner, to refer you to another specialist.
7. You have the right to see your medical records.

Your Responsibilities

1. Be assertive – ask, demand, tell, confront, refuse, persist, question, understand! You don't need to be aggressive – remember, the doctor is on your side!
2. Be well informed – join a self-help group. Read the currently available literature about your particular problem.
3. Keep your own record of all tests, results, and treatments.

4. Prepare a list of questions before you keep your appointment with the doctor. Also, write down the doctor's answers. If you wish to tape the interview, ask for the doctor's permission.
5. Take a long appointment if you feel you need more time with the doctor.
6. Inform the doctor or the receptionist if you are unable to attend a particular consultation.
7. Take your partner with you to the doctor — this can be mutually supportive.
8. Defer any treatment you are unsure about.
9. Do not have unreasonable expectations about your doctor. Understand that he may be tired, overworked, rushed or sick at times.
10. If you cannot communicate with your doctor, it is in your best interest to find someone you can talk to.
11. If you are dissatisfied with your treatment, try to discuss this aspect with the doctor and attempt to rectify the situation.
12. If you have unexplained infertility and all possible investigations and treatments have been tried, you may like to return to your doctor once in every two years to check on new developments in the field that may help you.

Emotional Care

When confronted by infertility, you need more than medical care; however, it is important to realize that your medical team is not likely to be your emotional care team as well. If this is what you expect, your frustration will be intensified. Your emotional support team could include relatives, friends, counsellors or infertility support groups.

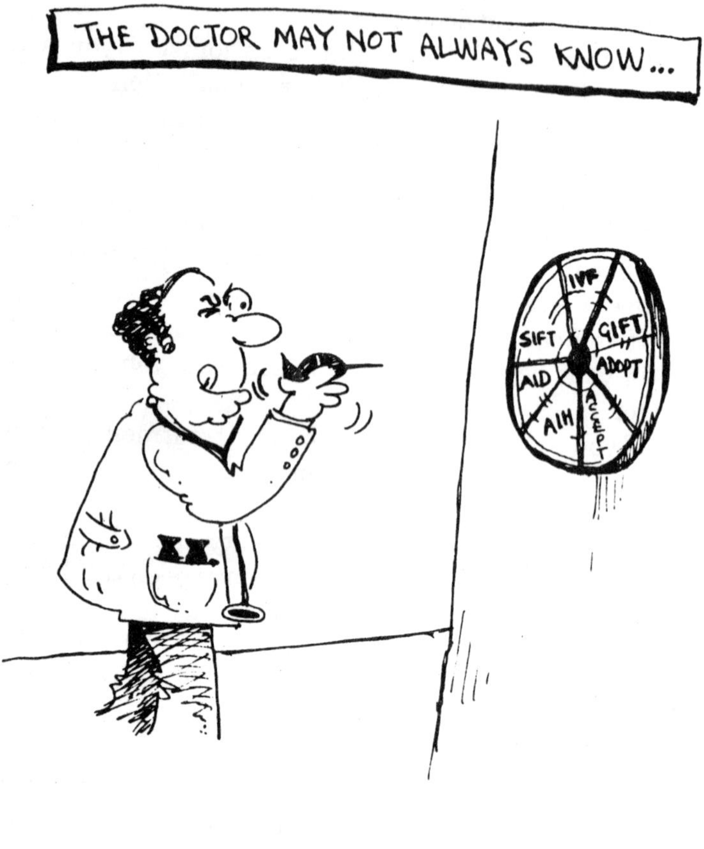
THE DOCTOR MAY NOT ALWAYS KNOW...
IVF
SIFT
GIFT
ADOPT
AID
AIH
ACCEPT

37

The Ethical Issues – Right or Wrong?

THE NEW REPRODUCTIVE TECHNOLOGIES have spawned a whole lot of new ethical concerns. These subjects are controversial ones, which have attracted wide media attention and public debate. However, the law and public opinion all over the world have lagged behind the rapid advances in artificial conception which have created a "brave new world" of possibilities of giving birth, never before considered possible, by using a mix-and-match combination of sperm, eggs and uteri.

Artificial conception raises the possibilities of myriad problems, legal or otherwise, which may need resolution by legislation or national guidelines. These problems relate to:

- The question of embryo research and the time limits to be placed on it. Basic questions such as – when does life begin? and what are the rights of an embryo? – remain unanswered.
- Guidelines on semen banking.
- The child's right of access to information about his/her genetic background and mode of conception.
- The legality of surrogacy
- The registration and monitoring of IVF clinics to ensure that infertile couples are not exploited.

Theologians the world over differ sharply on the subject. For example, to the Catholic Church, adoption is acceptable, as are the use of fertility drugs. GIFT procedures are allowed when the sperm and eggs of the couple are placed in the woman's own fallopian tubes. However, surrogacy, artificial insemination by husband or donor, and IVF are not allowed, because procreation without sexual union in considered unnatural, and the Church has been quite vocal in its criticism.

In Judaism, donor insemination is forbidden because a child is considered to be the offspring of the biological father only. Artificial insemination using the husband's sperm and IVF are accepted when there is a need to treat the disorder of infertility.

Most individuals have their own personal beliefs and convictions regarding the "rightness" or otherwise of many of the aforementioned techniques. Many people believe that embryos should not be used for research because they have the potential to become human beings, and, in fact, embryo research is banned in Germany by law.

Others feel that to restrict research is unfair to infertile couples, who should be allowed to make their own choices.

There will always be two points of views regarding the technology of assisted conception. At one end of the spectrum, will be people who feel that this technology allows couples to manipulate Nature artificially in order to produce children and will object to it. At the other end, will be people who believe that this technology represents a triumph of man's ingenuity which can be used to overcome Nature's constraints. It will never be possible to reconcile these two conflicting viewpoints since each of them is based on deeply held personal beliefs (and not facts), and we will have to learn to live with this moral dichotomy. At least, this clash of beliefs emphasizes the significance of the heated debates about when life begins! Since it may never be possible to have a consensus on this issue, this decision should not be left to moralists, or to philosophers, or to governments, or to doctors. Instead, the decision should be left to each individual couple, who ultimately provide the reproductive apparatus to create the baby.

Remember, there are no "right" or "wrong" answers — you must follow your own conscience.

38

How Much Does Treatment Cost?

BEING INFERTILE CAN PROVE TO BE A very expensive proposition! The various tests and courses of treatment needed cost considerable money, and since there is no definite end-point, budgeting for medical expenses can be very difficult.

The availability of modern assisted reproductive techniques, such as IVF, has made treatment even more expensive, since a great deal of medical expertise and scientific technology are needed for these procedures. This means that there really is no upper limit to how much you can spend in your pursuit of a baby!

You need to control your finances -- and it is unfortunately only too common to find patients who are so desperate to have a baby, that they have begged and borrowed, and even sold their lands, possessions and belongings, so that they could continue trying to have a baby.

Of course, for infertile couples, a baby is priceless, but you cannot afford to waste money. You may need to "shop around" to get a realistic estimate of how much the treatment actually costs. Charges vary widely, and don't automatically assume that the more expensive a clinic is, the better it is!

HOW MUCH DOES TREATMENT COST?

It is important to get a breakdown of the expenses for all procedures, from the doctor or clinic, preferably in writing. For example, for surgery, find out what exactly is included in the quoted figure – does it include just the surgeon's fees? the assistant's? anesthesia? operation theatre charges? hospitalization charges? followup visits? Often what is excluded can add up to a pretty large sum! This is especially true for IVF treatment, where "hidden expenses" can lead to your spending much much more than you had bargained for.

Patients are often reluctant to talk about money and expenses with doctors. Remember, however, it's your hard-earned money that you are spending – don't throw it away! You can't afford to shy away from this topic. Doctors also sometimes tend to be vague about money matters, and this makes getting specific figures so much more important.

You need to calculate what your *total* expenses will be, not just the medical costs. Remember to include travelling costs, lodging and boarding costs if you are from out-of-town, and the cost of time taken off from work.

Unfortunately, most insurance companies in India will not reimburse you for the medical expenses incurred for treating infertility – these companies still cling to the old-fashioned view that infertility is not a medical problem! A number of couples are also reluctant to claim medical expenses for infertility treatment, since they do not wish to disclose their "secret problem" to anyone else. Also, government medical facilities rarely provide quality care for infertility, since this is not a primary concern for them. Until these attitudes change, a number of patients will be deprived of infertility care, because of financial constraints – and this is a shame !

Approximate costs for the various procedures, tests and treatments are summarized in the following chart. These figures are for 1993 for the city of Bombay, and are only meant to be representative – however, do remember there can be considerable variation in costs! These are "all-inclusive" medical expenses.

Initial consultation	Rs 250 to Rs 500
Semen analysis	Rs 100 to Rs 200
Hysterosalpingogram	Rs 500 to Rs 1000
Hormonal blood assays (FSH, LH prolactin, estrogen, progesterone)	Rs 200 to Rs 300 (for each test)
Testicular biopsy	Rs 2000 to Rs 5000
Endometrial biopsy	Rs 500 to Rs 2000
Diagnostic laparoscopy	Rs 3000 to Rs 7000
Operative laparoscopy	Rs 5000 to Rs 12,000
Major surgery (microsurgery for tubal repair)	Rs 10,000 to Rs 25,000
IUI (insemination)	Rs 3000 to Rs 5000
TID (therapeutic insemination by donor), per cycle	Rs 3000 to Rs 5000
HMG treatment cycle (for superovulation)	Rs 5000 to Rs 15,000
GIFT	Rs 25,000 to Rs 60,000
IVF	Rs 25,000 to Rs 60,000

Additional procedures such as embryo freezing and microinjection are much more expensive.

39

Pregnant – At Last!

FOR MOST INFERTILE PATIENTS, GETTING pregnant is the ultimate dream which keeps them going through tests, treatments and surgery. What happens when the dream finally comes true?

Making the Diagnosis of Pregnancy

How do you find out if you are pregnant? For most treatments, doctors will wait till you miss your period before starting pregnancy testing. Ask your doctor when you should schedule a pregnancy test every time you take treatment – after all, you never know when it's going to work! A reasonable choice would be to conduct the test 16 to 18 days after ovulation. For IVF and GIFT cycles, in some clinics, testing may start as early as 10 to 12 days after the embryo transfer or GIFT.

When the pregnancy test is positive, the first response is often one of disbelief since it's hard to believe you are finally pregnant, especially if you have been trying for many years. Some patients tend to get emotional – it's finally happened! The time and effort and money have paid off! Infertility is now only a memory! But you soon realize that it's not all over. What you want is not a pregnancy but a baby! There are still uncertainties, and things could still go wrong, which is why careful monitoring is essential.

A pregnancy should be documented as early as possible. This is important, because appropriate care and precautions can then be taken at an early stage. The most sensitive pregnancy test is a blood test for the presence of beta-HCG (human chorionic gonadotropin). The HCG is produced by the embryo, and serves as the embryo's signal to the mother that pregnancy has occurred.

HCG can be measured in the blood by RIA (radioimmunoassay) or ELISA (enzyme immunoassay) testing; and positive levels (more than 10 mIU/ml) in the blood can be detected as early as two days before the period is missed. In the old days, the only way of determining the presence of HCG was by testing the urine, i.e, by using urine pregnancy test kits. Modern urine pregnancy kits (using monoclonal antibody technology) are quite sensitive and can detect a pregnancy as early as one to two days after a period has been missed (at a blood HCG level of about 50 to 100 mIU/ml). The benefit of urine pregnancy test kits is that they are less expensive, and testing can be done at home by the patient herself. However, instructions need to be followed carefully, and errors in interpreting the test results are not uncommon. These errors could occur if the urine is too dilute, or if the test is not done properly, or if a urinary tract infection exists.

The major advantage of blood tests is the fact that they measure the actual level of the HCG in the blood – and this factor can be very helpful in managing pregnancy problems, if they occur. As the embryo grows rapidly, HCG levels normally double every two to three days. Thus, one reliable sign of a healthy pregnancy is the fact that the HCG levels are increasing rapidly, and often doctors may need to do two HCG level tests three days apart in order to determine the viability of the pregnancy. A rising HCG level is reassuring.

Problems with HCG testing can occur if you have earlier been given HCG (human chorionic gonadotropin) injections for inducing ovulation. Normally, this exogenous HCG is excreted by the body in 10 days, but sometimes it can linger on. This is why, if the HCG level is very low, the test may need to be repeated, to confirm that the level is increasing.

What are "biochemical pregnancies"? These are pregnancies in which the HCG test is positive after the period has been missed; the levels increase, but are still low; and no pregnancy is ever documented on ultrasound. Biochemical pregnancies are often seen after IVF and GIFT. While they are not clinical pregnancies, they are of useful prognostic information, because they may mean that your chances of getting pregnant in a future cycle are good.

One drawback with the HCG test is that a positive HCG simply means a pregnancy is present in the body; it does not provide any information about the location of this pregnancy, which may be tubal or ectopic.

During the very early stages of pregnancy, HCG levels are the only way of monitoring the pregnancy. HCG levels which do not increase as rapidly as they should may mean that there is a problem with the pregnancy – the embryo may miscarry because it is unhealthy, or the pregnancy could be an ectopic pregnancy. Differentiating between the two conditions is obviously important, and this is where vaginal ultrasound plays a key role.

With vaginal ultrasound, it is possible to detect a pregnancy as early as two to four days after a missed period. An early pregnancy is observed as a pregnancy sac (also called a gestational sac) in the uterine cavity. The uterine lining is thick and bright white, and the sac appears as a black bubble in this lining. The sac should grow (at the rate of about 1 mm per day), and, if it does so, this is reassuring. The sac represents only the placental tissue – the embryo is so tiny at this stage, that it cannot be seen on ultrasound. At six weeks of pregnancy, an echo can be seen within the sac; this is the embryo. This embryo grows rapidly, so that on scans done at eight weeks, one should be able to see a beating fetal heart as well. This is very good evidence of a healthy fetus and the chances of a problem occurring in pregnancy after this point are small.

Ultrasound is useful because it provides information about not only the number of pregnancies (multiple pregnancies are not uncommon after infertility treatment and should be looked for!) but also their location. If the sac is not seen in the uterine cavity, then a tubal pregnancy should be suspected. The ultrasound provides information which is complementary to that of the HCG level. Often, both tests need to be done simultaneously and the results interpreted together.

What about do's and don'ts during pregnancy? What precautions should you take to minimize your risks? Unfortunately, there is little anyone can do today which is of much use. During pregnancy, most doctors may put you on supplemental progesterone injections (to help support the endometrium); and perhaps may recommend multi-vitamins, and low-dose aspirin. All this treatment is empiric — there is no proof that it really works! Also, many patients will put themselves on bed rest to prevent disturbing the pregnancy and the value of such rest is doubtful as well. If the pregnancy is going to encounter a problem, no matter what you do, it will. And if it is going to be uneventful, then you don't really need medical attention in any case. The trouble is that nobody knows which pregnancy is going to face problems and which one is not! During pregnancy, any bleeding, no matter how slight, should be taken seriously — and usually calls for hospitalization.

Unfortunately, it is a fact of life that 10% to 20% of all pregnancies will end in a miscarriage, and the risk of miscarriage in infertile women is even higher. This is because they are often older; or the medical problems which caused their infertility can also cause miscarriage, or sometimes the infertility treatment also increases this risk. Of course, some of the increased risk is only apparent, because the testing is so intensive and thorough.

Unfortunately, no treatment exists for preventing early miscarriages, and all that the doctor (and patient) can do is wait and watch. This suspense can be shattering! Nevertheless, the fact that you have got pregnant provides hope for the future.

If the pregnancy miscarries, then a curettage is needed. The tissue removed by curettage must be sent for histopathologic examination, in order to provide documentation of the pregnancy. This examination also helps to rule out an ectopic pregnancy.

Coping with a miscarriage after a long duration of infertility treatment can be pure hell! When you finally get pregnant after so many years of trying, you feel it is cruel on god's part to then snatch the baby away. In fact, perhaps the only trauma worse than not being able to conceive is to lose a pregnancy after trying so hard. Remember that neither Nature is perfect, nor is medical care. The most painstaking attention to detail cannot stop the unexpected from happening and no amount of obsession with detail will guarantee a perfect outcome.

If you miscarry, you are going to blame yourself — that it was something you did (or did not do) which caused the miscarriage. However, remember that 70% of miscarriages are because of a chromosomal abnormality at conception — something over which you have no control.

We will never know the reason why most miscarriages occur. This is why most doctors would not investigate you after just one miscarriage, since the chance of finding something significantly abnormal is so small, and your chance of having a healthy pregnancy the next time is better than 85%. Most doctors would reassure you, and the best option would be to try again (even though this can be emotionally very taxing!). If you've had a previous miscarriage, it is very normal to be frightened and worried, and restarting infertility treatment can be very difficult. You have to start from scratch all over again, and you wonder if and when you will again get pregnant. The lurking fear of losing the pregnancy once more, if you do conceive again, could torment you as well.

Coping with pregnancy after infertility treatment can be difficult even if the pregnancy is progressing normally. A great deal of time, energy, love and money has been invested in the pregnancy, and you don't want to take the slightest chance that something will go wrong. The anxiety can be overpowering, and even the minor aches and pains of pregnancy can send you rushing to the doctor for reassurance that all is well.

Your pregnancy should be monitored carefully, and this may involve frequent visits to the doctor, as well as repeated ultrasound scans. You will be very vulnerable and terrified, and will be bombarded by suggestions from well-meaning friends and relatives as to what to do, and also what not to do.

If you are more than 35 years of age, your doctor may advise you to undergo a chorion biopsy or amniocentesis in order to screen for genetic defects in the fetus, such as Down's syndrome. Also, if you have multiple pregnancies, frequent hospitalization and bed rest may be needed.

Yours is a "premium pregnancy", and will be treated as such even though your risk of developing complications is no more than any other woman's. However, since the pregnancy is so precious, the hazard is greater than for someone has no trouble conceiving, which is why an "at risk" approach to managing your pregnancy is appropriate. These factors greatly increase the chance of your requiring a caesarean section for birth, because neither you nor your doctor will want to take the slightest "chance" of something going wrong.

What happens after the delivery? Is this when the joy and happiness you have been anticipating for so long begin? Maybe! Certainly life is never the same when the child you have been looking forward to for so long finally arrives, especially if you have delivered twins! Babies are very demanding and not everyone can adjust easily to the new situation. If couples are older, then it may be harder for them to cope with the changes, especially after spending years of being together without the company of children.

The infertile woman who becomes pregnant expects perfection in every aspect of motherhood, because that's the stuff dreams are made of. However, when the reality of pregnancy, delivery and parenting actually takes hold, you may even feel disappointed, because real life is often harsher and unkinder than you had imagined. For example, you may have a hard time coping with 2 a.m. feedings and you may even start to resent your having to get up to take care of your newborn. This can make you feel guilty for not appreciating what you have – your child, for which you worked so hard! Don't worry, this feeling is normal and will pass.

Your parenting also is going to be influenced by your experience of infertility, because your child is extraspecial and it is natural for you to want to dote on him or her. This can be wonderful for your child because he or she will always know how much he or she was wanted and how much he or she is loved; but watch out for the emotional traps of being overprotective and unintentionally spoiling the child.

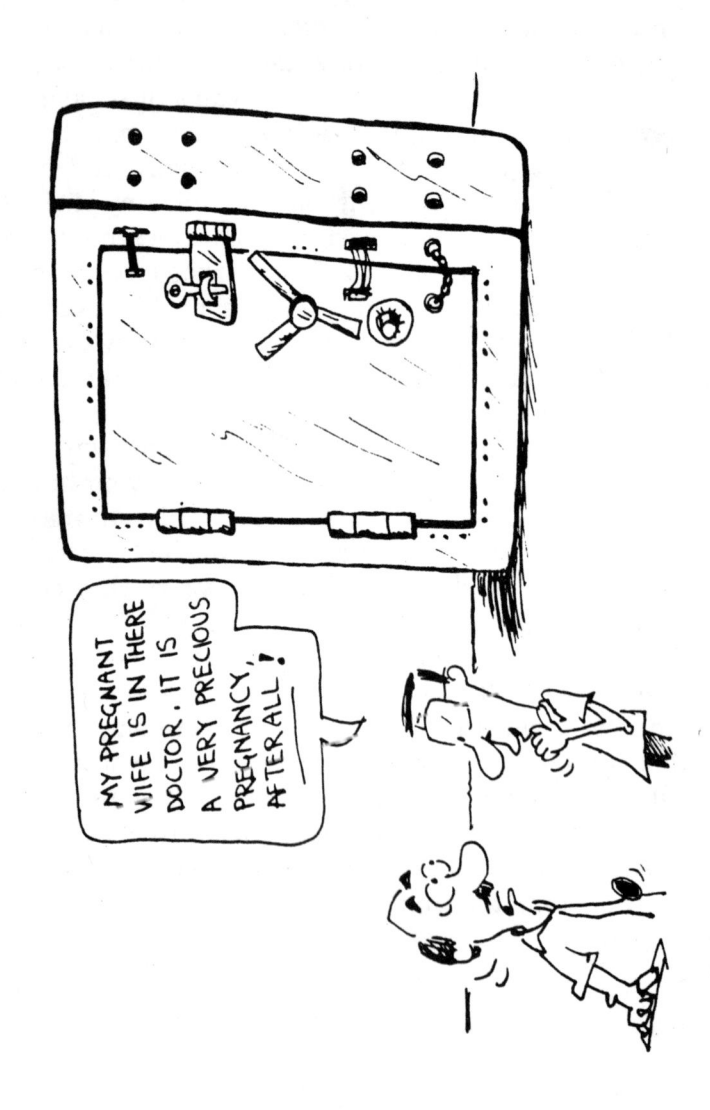

288　　　GETTING PREGNANT– A GUIDE FOR THE INFERTILE COUPLE

40

Preventing Infertility

PREVENTING INFERTILITY IS MUCH EASIER and better than treating it! This chapter outlines what you can do to reduce the risk of being infertile.

The biggest preventable danger to fertility is caused by uncontrolled sexually transmitted diseases (STDs) such as syphilis, gonorrhea and chlamydia and now AIDS as well. These diseases can cause irreparable damage to the reproductive tract in both men and women. STDs can usually be prevented by:

- Being thoroughly informed about STDs and by being aware of the risks they pose.
- Not engaging in promiscuous sexual activity. Abstinence or monogamy is the safest option!
- Using condoms if there is more than one sexual partner.
- Testing (for STD) if you feel you are at risk.
- Taking early and thorough treatment for STDs. This includes: careful followup; testing for cure; and screening of sexual partners.

Often, couples will want to postpone child bearing after marriage, and use contraceptives for this. Contraception can also pose a hazard to future fertility, if not selected carefully. For instance:

- IUDs should not be used in women who face an increased risk of developing STDs, because they increase the risk of pelvic inflammatory disease. It may be a good idea not to use IUDs at all in women who have never conceived.
- Oral contraceptives usually have no direct effect on fertility at all. However, women who have irregular anovulatory cycles before taking the pill will find that their irregular cycles return once they stop the pill and they may need treatment for this disorder.
- The use of depot contraceptives (such as Norplant) can interfere with the resumption of ovulation, leading to infertility.
- Sterilization (tubal ligation and vasectomy) as a method of family planning should be offered only to those couples who are sure they have completed their families; have received adequate counselling; and whose children have grown up.

An important preventable cause of testicular damage in men relates to uncorrected undescended testes. Such testes should be surgically treated at a very early age, to prevent them suffering damage as a result of exposure to body temperature, preferably before the age of two years. This requires educating mothers of young boys, and doctors as well.

It may also be a good idea to immunize boys against mumps in childhood, thus preventing the ravages which this disease can cause to the testes later in life.

Many "recreational" drugs – including alcohol, cocaine and marijuana – are poisons. They can reduce the sex drive, damage the sperm production, and interfere with ovulation; and sometimes such damage is irreparable. Smoking tobacco also affects the reproductive function – by depleting egg production, increasing the risk of PID (pelvic inflammatory disease), and lowering sperm counts.

Often, the adverse effect is temporary, so that when one stops taking these drugs, their harmful effects on the reproductive function are likely to be reversed. However, since abstinence is easier than moderation, the best option is not to smoke, drink or use drugs!

Occupational hazards can also decrease sperm counts. Many toxic drugs – including radiation, radioactive materials, anesthetic gases, and industrial chemicals (such as lead, the pesticide DBCP and the pharmaceutical solvent ethylene oxide) – can reduce fertility by impairing sperm production. Intense exposure to heat in the workplace (for example, long-distance truck drivers exposed constantly to engine heat, and men working in furnaces or in bakeries) can cause long-term and even permanent impairment of sperm production. You should be aware of these hazards and may need to control your exposure if infertility poses a problem.

Wearing loose cotton underwear and trousers is advisable – tight clothes increase testicular temperature and may harm sperm production.

X-rays can be harmful to gonads. If X-rays are needed at all, the scrotum should be covered with a lead shield.

Unnecessary surgery can also cause harm to fertility. For example, appendectomy for chronic abdominal pain in young women can create pelvic adhesions which damage the tubes. It is also important to educate doctors and patients about the necessity (or the non-necessity!) of certain operations in young women. Procedures like ovarian cystectomy to remove small ovarian cysts; myomectomy to remove small fibroids; and D&Cs may actually lead to more harm than do good. If surgical procedures are really needed, then these should be performed meticulously, preferably using microsurgical techniques. At present, minimally invasive surgery (laparoscopic surgery and ultrasound-guided procedures) offers an alternative to conventional surgery in those patients for whom conserving fertility is a major concern.

For some young men suffering from different forms of cancer (such as Hodgkin's lymphoma or testicular cancer), the therapy used for the cancer (chemotherapy and radiation) can destroy sperm production and render them sterile. For these men, sperm preservation (by freezing in a sperm bank) is an option they can choose in order to preserve their fertility.

Some young couples resort to abortions as a method of family planning when the women inadvertently get pregnant – either very soon after marriage or even before. These unwanted pregnancies are then removed by medical termination of pregnancy (MTP). An MTP is usually a safe and easy surgical procedure but it can lead to certain complications. One of these complications is infertility, resulting due to blocked tubes following an infection after surgery. Simple methods of contraception should be made easily available to couples, and they should be taught how to use them effectively.

It is also important to prevent unnecessary damage to the cervix in women. Regular Pap (cervical) smears to screen for early cervical precancerous disease allows conservative treatment of these lesions when they are found, thus preserving the function of the cervix. Unnecessary surgical treatment of benign cervical lesions such as erosions should also be avoided.

Young women who are obsessed with their physical fitness and body image can, paradoxically, impair their own fertility. Excessive dieting together with too much exercise in order to maintain a thin figure can actually cause irregular menstrual cycles and stop ovulation. This is especially common in women athletes, swimmers, gymnasts and dancers; and in women affected by anorexia nervosa. Simply regaining body weight can reverse their infertility.

Obesity can also interfere with ovarian function. Excessive fat disrupts normal hormonal production, causing abnormal ovulation. Reducing body weight down to normal can rectify the defect.

Another problem which has become more prevalent recently is the advanced age at which women are opting to have babies. Because of socio-economic pressures, women prefer to complete their education and pursue their careers before starting a family. This sometimes means that child bearing is postponed till women are in their late twenties or early thirties, and, for some women at least, the biological clock has ticked on too far as a result of this delay. In addition to the natural decline in fertility with increasing age, the longer a woman puts off pregnancy, the more she risks having her fertility threatened for various other reasons, such as endometriosis and STDs. While postponing child bearing can be an economic necessity for some couples, the best time to have a baby from a biological point of view is when the woman is in her early twenties.

41

The Infertile Patient's Prayer and Infertility "Defined"

Lord, give me strength...
To keep my cool when another period starts.
To keep my chin up when a relative announces her pregnancy.
To have a good relationship with my friend in spite of her ability to conceive easily and not be jealous of her.
To endure my sister-in-law's comments about toilet training!
To keep myself from crying when I see children begging on the roads.
To forgive my doctor when he keeps me waiting for hours for a consultation, and then can't remember my name!
To make the right decisions about treatment.
To maintain a good relationship with my husband in spite of all the trials and tribulations.

Infertility is...
Watching your husband playing with your friend's baby and wishing you could give him one of your own.
Telling nurses to please take blood from your right arm because the veins in your left arm are all exhausted because of all the IVs you've had!

Avoiding people you haven't seen for a long time because you don't want to hear the question: "Do you have any kids yet?"

Feeling very left out when your friends start comparing their pregnancy or child birth experiences.

Feeling like the whole town is pregnant except for you.

Getting tired of people always expecting you to do things for them, because "you don't have any kids to worry about".

Waking up in the middle of the night and wishing you could hear your baby crying.

Wishing you could give your parents grandchildren.

Wanting to fall apart if one other person says: "Why don't you adopt?"

Sometimes avoiding friends who are pregnant or with newborns because you just can't handle the situation at that moment.

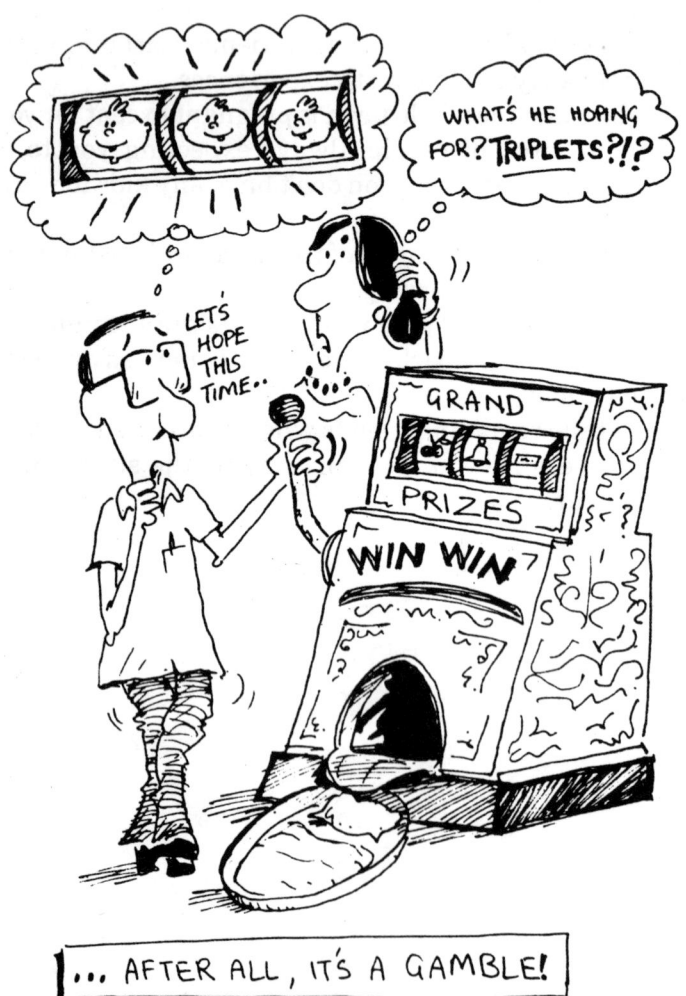

Appendix 1

Semen Analysis Chart

Name of patient	: ....
Date	: ....
Time specimen produced	: ....
Time analysis begun	: ....
Days since last ejaculation	: ....
Method of collection	: ....
Any spillage ?	: ....
Present medications	: ....

Parameter	Results/normal values
Colour	Gray
Coagulate?	Yes
Liquefy ?	Yes
If yes, time in minutes	< 30
Volume (ml)	2 to 6

(Appendix 1 cont'd.)

Parameter	Results/normal values
Viscosity	
pH	7.5 to 8.0
Sperm concentration (million per ml)	20 to 200
Grade of sperm motility	Grade 3,4
% motility	> 60%
Motile sperm count	> 10
White blood cells	< 1
Agglutination	nil
Morphology	> 50%

Appendix 2

Normal Hormone Values

Men

Testosterone	:	300 to 1100 ng/dl
Prolactin	:	7 to 18 ng/ml
Luteinizing hormone (LH)	:	2 to 18 mIU/ml
Follicle-stimulating hormone (FSH)	:	2 to 18 mIU/ml
Estradiol	:	< 60 pg/ml

Women

Hormone	Phase of cycle		
	Follicular	Day of LH surge	Midluteal
Luteinizing hormone (LH)	< 7 mIU/ml	>15 mIU/ml	—
Follicle-stimulating hormone (FSH)	< 13 mIU/ml	>15 mIU/ml	
Estradiol	—	> 100 pg/ml	
Progesterone	—	<1.5 ng/ml	> 15 ng/ml

(Appendix 2 cont'd.)

Prolactin	< 25 ng/ml
Thyroid-stimulating hormone (TSH)	0.4 to 3.8 µIU/ml
Free T3 (Triiodothyronine)	1.4 to 4.4 pg/ml
Free T4 (Thyroxine)	0.8 to 2.0 ng/dl
Total testosterone	6.0 to 86 ng/dl
Free testosterone	0.7 to 3.6 pg/ml
DHEAS (Dehydroepiandrosterone sulphate)	35 to 430 ug/dl
Androstenedione	0.7 to 3.1 ng/ml

Glossary

Abortion: The medical term for miscarriage. The various types of abortion include:
Complete abortion: A miscarriage in which all the products of conception have been expelled and the cervix is closed.
Habitual abortion: A miscarriage occurring on two or more separate occasions.
Incomplete abortion: A miscarriage in which only a portion of the products of conception has been expelled. This usually requires dilatation and curettage.
Induced abortion: An intentional termination of pregnancy.
Inevitable abortion: A miscarriage that cannot be halted.
Missed abortion: A miscarriage in which a dead fetus and other products of conception remain in the uterus for four or more weeks.
Selective abortion: A term often used to refer to intentional termination of one or more pregnancies within the uterus, usually in the case of a multiple pregnancy (triplets or more).
Spontaneous abortion: A miscarriage or the unintended termination of a pregnancy before the twentieth week.
Therapeutic abortion: An intentional termination of pregnancy for the purpose of preserving the life of the mother.
Threatened abortion: This produces symptoms such as vaginal bleeding, with or without pain, which may end

either in a miscarriage, or with the continuation of a normal pregnancy.

Adhesion: An abnormal attachment of adjacent tissues by bands, scars or masses of fibrous tissue.

Adrenal glands: Two glands near the kidneys that produce hormones, including some male sex hormones, namely, the adrenal androgens.

Agglutination of sperm: Sticking together of sperm.

Amenorrhea: The absence of menstruation.

Ampulla: The outer half of the fallopian tube, where fertilization occurs. The ampulla opens into the abdominal cavity through the tubal ostium (opening), which is lined by the fimbria.

Androgens: Male sex hormones; testosterone is one example.

Andrology: The science of diseases peculiar to the male sex, particularly infertility and sexual dysfunction.

Anomaly: A malformation or abnormality in any part of the body.

Anovulation: Total absence of ovulation. (*Note*: This is not necessarily the same as "amenorrhea". Menses may still occur with anovulation.)

Anovulatory bleeding: The type of menstruation often associated with failure to ovulate; this menstruation may be scanty and of short duration, or abnormally heavy and irregular.

Antibody: A protective protein produced in the body that fights, or otherwise interacts with, a foreign substance in the body.

Artificial insemination by donor (AID): The injection of donor semen into a woman's reproductive tract for the purpose of conception.

Artificial insemination by husband (AIH): The injection of husband's semen into the wife's reproductive tract for the purpose of conception.

Aspermia: The absence of semen. (*Note*: This is not the same as azoospermia.)

GLOSSARY

Asthenospermia: A condition in which the sperm do not move (swim) at all or move more slowly than normal.

Azoospermia: The absence of sperm in the ejaculate.

Basal body temperature (BBT): The temperature of the woman, taken either orally or rectally, upon waking in the morning before any activity; used to help determine when ovulation has occurred.

Bicornuate uterus: A congenital malformation of the uterus in which it appears to have two "horns" (cornu).

Capacitation: The process by which sperm are altered (usually during their passage through the female reproductive tract) that gives them the capacity to penetrate and fertilize the ovum.

Cervix: The lower section of the uterus which protrudes into the vagina.

Child-free living: A resolution to infertility in which the couple opts for a life-style without parenting, either temporarily or permanently.

Chlamydia: A sexually transmitted disease that may cause impaired fertility.

Chromosomes: Rod-shaped bodies in a cell's nucleus which carry the genes that convey hereditary characteristics; made up of DNA.

Cilia: Microscopic hair-like projections from the surface of a cell capable of beating in a coordinated fashion.

Clitoris: The small erectile sex organ of the female, located in front of the vagina and similar to the penis of the male.

Clomiphene citrate: A synthetic drug used to stimulate the hypothalamus and the pituitary gland in order to increase FSH and LH production. This drug is usually used to treat ovulatory problems due to hypothalamic pituitary dysfunction.

Coitus: Sexual intercourse.

Conception: The fertilization of a woman's egg by a man's sperm resulting in a new life.

Congenital: A characteristic or defect present at birth. It is acquired during fetal life, but is not necessarily hereditary.

Corpus luteum: The special gland that is formed in the ovary at the site of the released egg. This gland produces the hormone progesterone during the second half of the normal menstrual cycle.

Cryobank: A place where tissues (i.e., sperm, oocytes, embryos) are stored in the frozen state.

Cryopreservation (freezing): A procedure used to preserve (by freezing) and store embryos or gametes (sperm, oocytes).

Cryptorchidism: Undescended testicles.

Dilatation and curettage (D & C): Dilatation of the cervix to allow scraping of the uterine lining with an instrument (curette). This is also a means to induce abortion in the first trimester of pregnancy.

Dysgenesis: Faulty formation of any organ.

Dysmenorrhea: Painful menstruation.

Dyspareunia: Painful intercourse for either the woman or the man.

Ectopic pregnancy: A pregnancy in which the fertilized egg is implanted at a site other than the uterine cavity (most commonly in the fallopian tube, but occasionally also in the ovary or the abdominal cavity).

Egg (oocyte) donation: Surgical removal of an egg from one woman for transfer into the fallopian tube or uterus of another woman.

Ejaculation: The male orgasm during which approximately 2 to 5 ml of semen (seminal fluid and sperm) is ejected from the penis.

Embryo: The term used to describe the early stages of fetal growth, from conception to the eighth week of pregnancy.

Embryo transfer: The introduction of an embryo into a woman's uterus after *in vitro* fertilization.

GLOSSARY

Endocrine system: The system of glands which produce hormones, including the pituitary, thyroid, adrenals, testicles and ovaries.

Endocrinologist: A doctor who specializes in diseases of the endocrine glands.

Endometrial biopsy: The extraction of a small sample of tissue from the uterus for examination; this biopsy is usually done to provide evidence of ovulation.

Endometriosis: The presence of endometrial tissue (the normal uterine lining) in abnormal locations such as the tubes, ovaries and peritoneal cavity, often causing painful menstruation and infertility.

Endometrium: The mucous membrane lining in the uterus.

Endosalpinx: The tissue lining in the fallopian tube.

Epididymis: An elongated organ in the male lying above and behind the testicles. It contains a highly convoluted canal, four to six metres in length, where, after production, sperm are stored, nourished and ripened for a period of several months.

Erection: The enlarged, rigid state of the penis when sexually aroused.

Estradiol (E2): A hormone released by developing follicles in the ovary. Plasma estradiol levels are used to help determine progressive growth of the follicle during ovulation induction.

Estrogen: A class of female hormones, produced mainly by the ovaries from the onset of puberty until menopause which are also responsible for the development of secondary sexual characteristics in women.

Fallopian tubes: A pair of narrow tubes that carry the ovum (egg) from the ovary to the body of the uterus.

Fertilization: The penetration of an egg by a sperm and the subsequent fusion of their genetic material, which results in the development of an embryo.

Fetal death: The term often used to include both miscarriage and still-birth.

Fetus: The developing baby from the ninth week of pregnancy until the moment of birth.

Fibroid tumour (leiomyoma): A benign tumour of fibrous tissue that may occur in the uterine wall; it may be totally without symptoms or may cause abnormal menstrual patterns or infertility.

Fimbriae: The fringed and flaring outer ends of the fallopian tubes which capture the egg after it is released from the ovary.

Follicle: The structure in the ovary that has nurtured the ripening egg and from which the egg is released.

Follicle-stimulating hormone (FSH): A hormone produced in the pituitary gland that stimulates the ovary to ripen a follicle for ovulation.

Follicular phase: The first half of the menstrual cycle when follicle development takes place in the ovary.

Frigidity: The inability to become sexually aroused; this condition is not a known cause of infertility.

Gamete: The male or female reproductive cell — the sperm or the ovum (egg), respectively.

Gamete intrafallopian transfer (GIFT): A procedure in which the sperm and eggs are transferred into the fallopian tubes (usually by laparoscopy) where fertilization may then take place.

Genes: Substances that convey hereditary characteristics, consisting primarily of DNA and proteins and occurring at specific points on the chromosomes.

Genetic: A term pertaining to hereditary characteristics.

Genetic abnormality: A disorder arising from an anomaly in the chromosomal structure which may or may not be hereditary.

Genetic counselling: Advice and information provided, usually by a team of experts, on the detection and risk of recurrence of genetic disorders.

Gestation: The period of fetal development in the uterus from conception to birth, which is usually 40 weeks in humans.

Gland: A hormone-producing organ.

GnRH (gonadotropin-releasing hormone; LHRH): A hormone released from the hypothalamus that controls the synthesis and release of the pituitary hormones, FSH and LH.

Gonadotropins: Hormones capable of stimulating the gonads to produce hormones and/or gametes. They are FSH and LH.

Gonads: The glands that produce the gametes (the testicles in the male and the ovaries in the female).

Gynecologist: A doctor who specializes in the diseases of the female reproductive system.

Hamster test (sperm penetration assay): A test used to determine the ability of a man's sperm to penetrate a hamster egg. Thought to provide evidence of the sperm's fertilizing ability.

Hemorrhage: Excessive bleeding.

Hereditary: Transmitted from one's ancestors by way of the genes within the chromosomes of the fertilizing sperm and egg.

Hirsutism: The presence of excessive body and facial hair, especially in women.

Hormone: A chemical, produced by an endocrine gland, which circulates in the blood and has widespread action throughout the body.

Human chorionic gonadotropin (HCG): A hormone secreted by the placenta during pregnancy that prolongs the life of the corpus luteum.

Human menopausal gonadotropin (HMG): A product containing both human FSH and LH. These hormones are extracted from the urine of postmenopausal women.

Hydrocele: A swelling in the scrotum containing fluid.

Hydrosalpinx: A large fluid-filled, club-shaped fallopian tube closed at the fimbriated end; it is a cause of infertility.

Hydrotubation: Lavage or "flushing" of the fallopian tubes with a sterile solution which sometimes contains medication such as antibiotics, enzymes or steroids.

Hymen: A membrane that partially covers the virgin vagina.

Hyperplasia: Abnormal enlargement of an organ or tissue of the body.

Hyperstimulation syndrome: A syndrome which may occur after the development of many eggs (superovulation); symptoms include ovarian enlargement, abdominal distension and weight gain.

Hypogonadism: Inadequate gonadal function as manifested by deficiencies in sperm production in males or egg production in females and/or the secretion of gonadal hormones (estrogens and androgens, respectively).

Hypospadias: A malformation of the penis in which the urethral opening is found on the underside rather than at the tip of the penis.

Hypothalamus: A part of the base of the brain that controls the release of hormones from the pituitary.

Hysterosalpingogram (HSG): An X-ray study in which a contrast dye is injected into the uterus to show the delineation of the body of the uterus and the patency of the fallopian tubes. Also called a tubogram or uterotubogram.

Idiopathic (unknown or unexplained): The term used when no reason can be found to explain the cause of a medical condition.

Immunological response: The production of antibodies (and other products) by the immune system, when activated as a result of exposure to a foreign substance.

Implantation: The embedding of the fertilized egg in the endometrium of the uterus.

Impotence: The inability of the male to achieve or maintain an erection for intercourse due to physical or emotional problems.

Incompetent cervix: A weakened cervix that is incapable of holding the fetus within the uterus for the full nine months; this can be a cause of late miscarriage.

Infertility: The inability of a couple to achieve a pregnancy after one year of regular unprotected sexual intercourse, or the inability of the woman to carry a pregnancy to live birth.

Interstitial cells: The cells between the seminiferous tubules of the testicles that produce the male hormone testosterone. Also called Leydig cells.

In vitro (literally, in glass) fertilization (IVF): A procedure in which an egg is removed from a ripe follicle and fertilized by a sperm cell outside the human body. Also called "test tube baby" and "test tube fertilization".

In vivo fertilization: The fertilization of an egg by a sperm within the woman's body.

Kallman's syndrome: Hypogonadism with anosmia (loss of the sense of smell); uncommon cause of male infertility.

Karyotype: A study of the chromosomes of the tissue; used for genetic studies.

Klinefelter's syndrome: A congenital abnormality of the male wherein he receives an XXY chromosomal complement instead of XY. Such a man is infertile.

Labia: Folds of skin on either side of the entrance of the vagina.

Laparoscopy: The direct visualization of the ovaries and the exterior of the fallopian tubes and uterus by means of inserting a surgical telescope through a small incision below the navel.

Laparotomy: Abdominal surgery.

Leydig cells: *See* interstitial cells.

LHRH: Luteinizing hormone-releasing hormone (*see also* GnRH).

Libido: Sexual desire.

Luteal phase: The days of the menstrual cycle following ovulation and ending with menses during which progesterone is produced by the corpus luteum.

Luteal phase defect: A shortened luteal phase or one with inadequate progesterone production.

Luteinized unruptured follicle (LUF) syndrome: A condition in which the egg is not released during ovulation; the follicle does not rupture and the egg is trapped.

Luteinizing hormone (LH): A hormone secreted by the pituitary gland. Secretion of LH increases in the middle of the cycle to induce release of the egg.

Menarche: The onset of menstruation in girls.

Menopause: The cessation of menstruation in women due to aging or failure of the ovaries; most commonly occurs between the ages of 40 and 50.

Menotropins (human menopausal gonadotropin or HMG): Injections which contain the hormones FSH and LH; these injections are manufactured by extracting the hormones from the urine of menopausal women.

Menstruation: The shedding of the uterine lining by cyclic bleeding that normally occurs about once a month in the mature female.

Miscarriage: A spontaneous abortion of a fetus up to the age of fetal viability, i.e., 20 weeks of pregnancy.

Mittelschmerz: German word for "middle pain", referring to the pain that some women experience during ovulation.

Morphology of sperm: The study of the shape of sperm cells. This evaluation is part of a semen analysis.

Motility of sperm: The ability of the sperm to move about.

Mumps orchitis: Inflammation of the testicle caused by the mumps virus; this can lead to sterility if infection with the virus occurs after puberty.

Myomectomy: Surgical removal of a fibroid tumour (myoma) in the uterine muscular wall.

Necrospermia: A condition in which sperm are produced and found in the semen, but they are dead. Such sperm cannot fertilize eggs.

Nidation: The implantation of the fertilized egg in the endometrium of the uterus.

Obstetrician: A doctor who specializes in pregnancy and child birth.

Oligo-ovulation: Infrequent ovulation, usually less than six ovulatory cycles per year.

Oligospermia: An abnormally low number of sperm in the ejaculate of the male.

Oocyte (ovum): The egg.

Oocyte retrieval: A surgical procedure to collect the eggs contained within the ovarian follicles, usually done under ultrasound guidance.

Orchitis: An inflammation of the testes.

Ovarian failure: The inability of the ovary to respond to any gonadotropic hormone stimulation, usually due to the absence of oocytes.

Ovaries: The sexual gland of the female which produces the hormones estrogen and progesterone, and in which the ova are developed.

Oviduct. The fallopian tube.

Ovulation: The discharge of a mature egg, usually around the midpoint of the menstrual cycle.

Ovulation induction: The use of hormone therapy (clomiphene citrate, HMG,HCG) to stimulate oocyte development and release.

Ovum: The egg (reproductive) cell produced in the ovaries each month. (The plural of "ovum" is "ova".)

Pelvic inflammatory disease (PID): Inflammatory disease of the pelvis, often caused by infection.

Penis: The male organ of intercourse.

Pituitary: A gland located at the base of the human brain that secretes a number of important hormones related to normal growth, development and fertility.

Polycystic ovarian syndrome (PCOS): Development of multiple cysts in the ovaries due to arrested follicular growth, perhaps as a result of an imbalance in the amount of LH and FSH produced.

Polyp: A nodule or small growth found frequently on mucous membranes, such as in the cervix or the uterus.

Postcoital test (the Huhner test): A diagnostic test for infertility in which vaginal and cervical secretions are obtained following intercourse and then analysed under a microscope.

Progesterone: A hormone secreted by the corpus luteum of the ovary after ovulation has occurred; it is also produced by the placenta during pregnancy.

Prostate: A gland in the male that surrounds the first portion of the urethra near the bladder. It secretes an alkaline liquid that neutralizes the acid in the urethra and stimulates motility of the sperm.

Pyospermia: A condition in which the presence of white cells in the semen indicates possible infection.

Retrograde ejaculation: Discharge of semen backward into the bladder rather than forward through the penis.

Retroverted uterus: A uterus that is bent backward; not a cause of infertility.

Rubin test: An obsolete test in which a gas such as carbon dioxide is blown into the uterus under pressure to test if the fallopian tubes are open.

Salpingitis: Inflammation of the fallopian tubes.

Salpingolysis: Surgery to clear the fallopian tubes of adhesions.

Salpingoplasty: Surgery to correct blocked fallopian tubes.

Scrotum: The bag of skin and thin muscle that holds the testicles.

Secondary infertility: The inability to conceive or carry a pregnancy after having successfully conceived and carried one or more pregnancies.

Semen: The sperm and seminal secretions ejaculated during orgasm.

Semen analysis: The study of a fresh ejaculate under the microscope.

Seminal vesicles: A pair of pouch-like glands above the prostate in the male that produce a thick, alkaline secretion that is passed in the semen during ejaculation.

Seminiferous tubules: The long tubes in the testicles in which sperm are formed.

Septum: An abnormality in organ structure present since birth in which a wall is present where one should not exist.

Sexually transmitted diseases (STD): Infections pertaining to, or transmitted during, sexual intercourse. Also known as VD or venereal diseases. Most commonly gonorrhea, syphilis and chlamydia, and now, AIDS as well.

Sperm (spermatozoa): The male reproductive cell, which has measurable characteristics such as:

Count (or density): This refers to the number of sperm present.

Morphology: This refers to the form or shape of the sperm.

Motility: This refers to the percentage of sperm demonstrating any type of movement.

Viability: This refers to whether or not the sperm are alive.

Sperm bank: A place in which sperm (from donor or from husband) is stored in a frozen state for future use in artificial insemination.

Sperm washing: A technique that separates the sperm from the seminal fluid.

Spermatogenesis: The production of sperm within the seminiferous tubules.

Spinnbarkheit: The stretchability of cervical mucus.

Split ejaculate: A method of collecting a semen specimen so that the first half of the ejaculate is caught in one container and the rest in a second container. The first half usually contains the majority of the sperm.

Superovulation: A treatment method in which the growth of multiple eggs is stimulated, in order to enhance the woman's fertility potential.

Surrogate mother: A woman who gestates a fetus and then turns over the child to the infertile couple, who may be its genetic parents.

Testicles: The male sexual glands, of which there are two. Contained in the scrotum, they produce the male hormone testosterone and produce the male reproductive cells, namely, the sperm.

Testicular biopsy: Surgical excision of testicular tissue to determine the ability of the testes to produce normal sperm.

Testicular failure: A condition in which the testes fail to produce sperm.

Testosterone: The most potent male sex hormone, produced in the testicles.

Test tube baby: A child born through *in vitro* fertilization.

Thyroid gland: A gland located at the front base of the neck which secretes the hormone thyroid that is necessary for normal fertility.

Tuboplasty: Surgical repair of fallopian tubes.

GLOSSARY

Turner's syndrome (ovarian dysgenesis): A congenital abnormality of the female wherein she receives an XO instead of an XX genetic sex complement. Women with this condition are infertile.

Ultrasound (sonography): An imaging technique which uses high-frequency sound waves, and is useful for visualizing structures in the female pelvis. Commonly used to monitor the growth of ovarian follicles during infertility therapy.

Unexplained infertility: *See* idiopathic infertility.

Urethra: The tube that carries urine from the bladder to the outside. In men it also carries semen from the prostate to the point of ejaculation during intercourse.

Urologist: A doctor who specializes in diseases of the urinary tract in men and women, and the genital organs in men.

Uterotubogram: *See* hysterosalpingogram.

Uterus: The hollow, muscular organ in the woman that holds and nourishes the fetus until the time of birth.

Vagina: The birth canal opening in the woman extending from the vulva to the cervix of the uterus.

Vaginismus: A spasm of the muscles around the opening of the vagina, making penetration during sexual intercourse either impossible or very painful.

Varicocele: A varicose vein of the testicles, sometimes a cause of male infertility

Vas deferens: A pair of thick-walled tubes (about 45 cm long) in the male that lead from the epididymis to the ejaculatory duct in the prostate.

Vasectomy: Surgery to excise a part of the vas deferens in order to sterilize a man.

Vasogram: X-ray of the male reproductive tract.

Venereal diseases (VD): *See* sexually transmitted diseases.

Viscosity: Thickness of the semen.

Vulva: The external genitalia of the female.
Zygote: An embryo in the early development stage.
Zygote intrafallopian transfer (ZIFT): Transfer of a zygote into a fallopian tube (usually done by laparoscopy).

Index

Abdominal pain, 96-97
Abortion, 136, 292
  medical definition of, 137
  see also miscarriages
ACTH (adrenocorticotropic hormone)
    stimulation test, 115
Adoption
  myths and facts about, 214
Adoption agencies, 212-214
AIDS, 171, 194, 195, 280
Antiphospholipid antibodies, 142, 143
Antisperm antibodies, 48
Antisperm antibodies test
  role of, 34-35
Artificial insemination by husband
    (AIH), 162
  cost of performing, 168
  intrauterine insemination (IUI)
      method, 164, 165
  methods of performing, 164
  recent advances in, 166-167
  psychological issues in, 167
  sperm processing for, 166-167
  success rate of, 167-168
  usefulness of, 162-163

Bacteria as cause of infertility, 52
Balloon tuboplasty or cornual
    recanalization, 88
Basal body temperature (BBT) chart,
    93-94, 244
  instructions for, 93-94
Beta-HCG test, 125
Billing's (fertility awareness method),
    107

Biochemical pregancies, 283
Blood tests, 37-38, 96, 98
Bovine cervical mucus test, 35-36
Brown, Louise, 169

C T Scan, 115
Cervical crypts, 106
Cervical mucus, 96, 106-107
  Billing's method for, 96
  observation of, 107-108
  problems with, 108
  SCMC test, 111-112
  tests on, 108-109
  treatment of, 112
Chemotherapy, effects of, 52
Child-free life
  advantages of, 218
  factors related to, 219-220
  fears created by, 218
Chlamydia, problem of, 51
Chorion biopsy, 286
Clomiphene stimulated FSH level, 170
Cohen, Dr Jacques, 185
Corona cells, 3
Corpus luteum, 91, 93, 130
Cumulus oophorus, 4
Curettage, 95
  procedure for infertile patients,
      95-96

D & C (dilatation and curettage), 95-96
Doppler test, 43, 51
Drugs of abuse, 50
Duct blockage, 45-46

317

Ectopic pregnancy, 124
  blood test for, 125-126
  causes of, 124-125
  diagnosis of, 125-126
  meaning of, 124
  occurrence of, 124
  surgical treatment for, 127
  ultrasound-guided treatment for, 126-127
Ejaculation problem, 53
  treatment for, 54
Electroejaculation for spinal cord problems, 55
Embryo culture, 173-174
Embryo freezing, 176-177
Embryo research
  ban in Germany by law, 276
Embryo transfer, 174-175
Endometrial biopsy, 26, 94-95
Endometriosis, 118
  causes of, 119
  diagnosis, of 121
  hormone medication treatment for, 122
  symptoms of, 119-120
  surgery treatment for, 123
Epididymis, 8, 9
Estrogen, 6
Ethical issues, 275
External genitals, 1
  openings of, 1

Fallopian tubes, 2, 19, 76, 80, 93
Falloposcopy method, 78, 85
Fertility potential of the couple
  concept of, 58
Fertility, reasons for downfall, 22
Fertilization process, 14-16
Female hormones, phases of, 5-7
Fimbriae, 80
Fluoroscopic guided procedures, 85
Follicle-stimulating hormone (FSH), 7, 37-38, 49, 103, 157, 172, 173

GIFT (gamete intrafallopion transfer), 48, 55, 56, 125, 132, 163, 169, 177-179, 202, 276, 283
  advantages of, 179
  and IVF compared, 179-180
  chances of achieving pregnancy with, 182-183
  cost of, 180
  disadvantages of, 180
  risks and complications of, 188-189
  use of donor sperm and eggs in, 187-188
  variations of, 180-181
GnRH (gonadotropin-releasing hormone), 7, 172, 173
Gonorrhea (effect on male genital tract), 51

Hair growth, types of, 133
  terminal, 113
  vellus, 113
Hepatitis B test, 171
Hirsutism
  ACTH test for, 115
  blood tests for, 115
  causes of, 113-114
  cosmetic therapy for, 116-117
  determining the cause of, 115
  treatment for, 115-116
HMG (human menopausal gonadotropin), 49, 154-157, 172
Hodgkin's disease, 52
Hormone imbalance, 48-49, 140
HCG (human chorionic gonadotropin), 49, 157, 282-283
HSG (hyrtersalpingogram),
  comparing laparoscopy and, 72-73,
  risks involved in, 84
Hyperprolactinemia problem, 49
Hysteroscopy, 76
  advantages of, 79
  as an important tool, 76
  operative, 77-78
  steps in, 76-77

Immunity problems, 141-142
Infections, 51, 131
  causes of, 51-52
Infertility
  coping with, in every day life, 232
  coping with treatment, 234
  cost of, 278-280
  definition of, 18, 136
  doctor-patient relationship, 246

INDEX

emotional signs of depression during, 239
ethical issues in, 275-277
effect on couple, 236-237
feelings about sexuality for the couple faced with, 242-243
investigation and diagnosis of, 243
lack of public support during, 247-248
medical factors, problems related to, 19-20, 223-227
medical tests for, 24-26
myths and misconceptions about, 252-256
prevention of, 289
psychological effects of, 241
regaining control during, 235-236
religious support during, 236
sharing your feelings during, 230-231
suggestions, 257-259
therapist advice for, 239-240
treatment programmes for, 246
unexplained, 129
Infertility Friends, address of, 250
Intercourse
 frequency of, 21
 position and technique of, 21-22
 timing of, 21
Interauterine insemination (IUI), 55, 56, 162-166
IUCD insertion, 124, 129
IVF (*in vitro* fertilization) 36-37, 46, 48, 55-57, 86, 90, 112,125, 132,169-172, 202, 246-247
 cost of, 175-176
 dramtic advance with regard to, 185-186
 pregancy rates due to, 183-184
 problems with, 185
 risks and complications of, 188-189
 use of donor sperm and eggs in, 187-188

Jabobs, Dr Howard, 141

Kerin, Dr John, 85

Klinefelter's syndrome, 40-41
Laparoscopy, 67
 abnormal findings during, 75
 and HSG, 84
 benefits of, 72
 comparing HSG and, 72-73
 diagnosis of many problems through, 67
 findings of, 74-75
 limitations of HSG and, 84-85
 operative, 70-71
 precautions before surgery, 68-69
 timing of, 67-68
Leukemia, 52
Lymphoma, 52
Luteal phase abnormalities, 130
Luteinizing hormone (LH), 7, 38, 91, 103, 157

Male infertility
 cause of, 59
 diagnosis of, 42
 medical warning for, 161-162
 tests for, 28, 57
 treatment for, 42
 medicines used in, 158-159
Male reproductive system, 7-11
Medical termination of pregnancy (MTP), 292
Medicines used (in infertility treatment), 148-160
Menopause, 247
Menstrual cycle, 5, 17
Menstrual period timing, 92-93
MESA (microepididymal sperm aspiration), 46
Miscarriages, 136, 284-286
 causes of, 138-140
 facts and fiction about, 138
 health problems as cause of, 140-141
 polycystic ovarian syndrome, cause of, 141
 problem of, 137
 term of, 136-137
 tests for, 145-146
 TORCH infections and, 141
 treatment for, 146-147
 uterine problems and, 143-144
Mittelschmerz (midcycle pain), 86

Natural cycle IVF, 186
Nocturnal penile tumescence (NPT) testing, 54
Normal hormone values, 299-300
Normal ovulation cycle, 92
  hormone changes in, 91-92

Occupation hazards as cause of infertility, 53
Orchitis, 51
Osler, Sir William, 223
Ovarian failure, 10
  treatment for, 101-102
Ovarian tumours, 114
Ovulation, 91
  abnormalities of, 99-100
  induction of, 104
Ovulation prediction test kits, 98-99

PID (pelvic inflammatory disease), 290
Polycystic ovarian disease (PCOD)/polycystic ovarian syndrome (PCOS) or Stein-Leventhal syndrome, 103
  diagnosis of, 103-104
  treatment for, 104-105
Postcoital test (PCT), 35, 109-110
Pregnancy test, 281-282
Primary infertility, 18
Premium pregnancy, 286
Progesterone, 5, 6

Radiation therapy, 52
Radioimmunoassay or ELISA test, 38
Ranoux, Dr Claude, 186
Rete testis, 9
Retrograde ejaculation, 54
  simple way to diagnose, 54-55
RT or Rubin's test, 81

Secondary infertility, 18, 133-135
Semen analysis, 28
  chart, 297-298
Semen culture test, 35, 51-52
Semen test for male, 28-33
Seminiferous tubules, 9
Silber, Dr Sherman, 46
Six treatment cycles, 58

Smallpox, 51
SONAR machines, 61
Sonosalpingography, 63, 85
Sperm cervical mucus contact test (SCMC), 111-112
Sperm immunity problems, 47
  treatment for, 48
Sperm penetration assay (SPA, hamster assay), 36-37
Sperm viability or sperm survival test, 36, 170
Sperm processing, 165-166
  laboratory techniques for, 166
STDs (sexually transmitted diseases), 51, 289, 290, 293
Sterilization, 90
  reversal of, 90
  why women regret, 90
Support groups, 248
  addresses of, 250-251
  misconceptions about, 249
Surrogacy, 201
  adverse publicity about, 203
  guidelines for, 202-203
  kinds of, 201-202
Syphilis, 51

Testes, undescended, 28, 50
Testicular biopsy, 39-41
Testicular tumours, 52
Testosterone, 12-13
Therapeutic insemination by donor (TID), 193
  advantages of frozen semen in, 199
  blood test for, 194-195
  common problems in, 198
  couples undergoing, 193-194
  disadvantages of fresh semen in, 199
  donor semen sample for, 194, 198
  mixing sperm during, 196
  treatment process during, 196-197
Tobacco as a cause of infertility, 50
TORCH test, 145
Torsion, 51
Transport IVF, 186-187
"Trying time"
  concept of, 58

INDEX

Tubal diseases, 81
   diagnosis of, 81-82
   HSG and, 82-83
   operative laparoscopy for repair, 89-90
   surgical treatment for, 86
Tubal damage, 87
   distal, 88
   proximal, 87
Tubal ligation, 90
Tubal microsurgery, 86-87
Tubal pregnancies, 124
Tubal reanastomosis, 88
Tubal repair, 89-90
   operative laparoscopy for, 89-90
Tuberculosis, 51
Tuboscopy method, 85

Ultrasound technology, 61
   advances in, 63-65
   advantages of, 64, 284
   by a radiologist, 62-63
   commonest use for, 61-62
   role of, 97
   scope of, 65
   uses in variety of problems, 64-65
Unexplained infertility, 129
   causes of, 130-131
   criteria for, 129
   diagnosis of, 129-130
   treatment of, 132

Varicocele, 42
   controversy regarding, 43
   conventional surgery for, 44
   diagnosis of, 43
   microsurgery method for, 44
   radiologic balloon occlusion for, 44-45
   reason for a low sperm count, 42-43
Vas deferens, 9, 46
Vasectomy, 47
Vasography, 40-41
Vasoepididymal anastomosis (VEA), 45
Vasovasostomy or VVA (vasovasal anastomosis), 47
VDRL (Venereal Diseases Research Laboratory), 145
Videolaparoscopy, 70

Woman's reproductive organs, 1-2

ZIFT, PROST or TET, 179
   see also, GIFT
Zona pellucida, 3